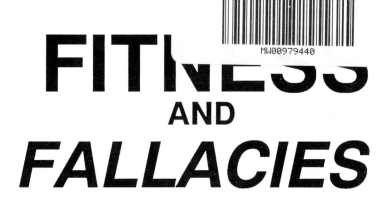

FITNESS
AND
FALLACIES

Everyone's Guide to Safe and Effective Exercise

Rick DeLorme, M.A., M.S.
Fred W. Stransky, Ph.D.
Meadow Brook Health Enhancement
Institute
Oakland University
Rochester, Michigan

Dr Cummings,
Thank You
For the wonderful Care!

Rick De

KENDALL/HUNT PUBLISHING COMPANY
4050 Westmark Drive   Dubuque, Iowa 52002

Dedicated to Fitness Instructors and Exercise Leaders Everywhere

Special thanks to the kind people at the Marguerite deAngeli Library, Lapeer, Michigan, where the first draft of this book was written.

I would like to express appreciation for the inspiration provided by Fred Stransky, my mentor, director and friend.

Rick DeLorme

Illustrations by Bonnie Miljour

Copyright © 1990 by Kendall/Hunt Publishing Company

ISBN 0-8403-5446-0

Printed in the United States of America
10 9 8 7

Contents

About Meadow Brook   **v**

Chapter 1
Exercise as an Industry   1

Chapter 2
The Myth of Body Toning   3
    Regional Exercise   **3**
    Spot Reduction   **4**
    Shaping, Sculpting and Toning   **4**
    Muscle Tonus   **6**
    The Cause of Undesirable Body Contours   **7**
    What Happens as a Person Becomes More
        Visibly Toned   **12**
    Acquiring the Toned Look   **13**
    How Can Tone be Measured Objectively?   **13**
    Body Composition   **14**
    Toning Tables and Electronic Stimulation   **17**
    The Fallacy of Body Toning: A Typical
        Scenario   **20**
    Chapter Summary   **20**

Chapter 3
**Exercise, Fitness and "Looking Good":
Getting the Most with a Limited
Amount of Time   23**
    The Benefits of Regular Exercise   **23**
    Components of Fitness   **25**
    The Development of Muscular Strength,
        Muscular Endurance, Muscle Size and
        Muscle Tone   **25**
    The Program   **27**
    Misconceptions of Muscular Hypertrophy   **30**
    The Physiology of "The Burn"   **36**

Cardiovascular Endurance: Aerobic
Capacity   **37**
Aerobic Exercise Prescription   **38**
Flexibility   **46**
Ballistic Stretching and the Stretch Reflex   **47**
Guidelines For Aerobic Exercise   **47**
Chapter Summary   **49**

Chapter 4

Safe Exercise: Screening for Those at Risk   51

Who Should Have a Maximal Exercise
Test?   **51**
Major Coronary Risk Factors   **52**
The Physical Activity Readiness
Questionnaire   **53**
Screening Procedure   **53**
Health and Exercise Risk Appraisal   **57**

Chapter 5

**Recommended and Contraindicated
Exercises   59**

Chapter 6

Fallacies of Exercise   75

Chapter 7

**Quality of Life and Body
Composition: The Nutrition Connection   85**

The Energy Balance Equation   **85**
Foods Generally High in Fat   **86**
Foods Generally High in Carbohydrate   **87**
Comparing Starchy and Fatty Foods   **88**
Disease Prevention   **88**
Dietary Recommendations   **89**
The Set Point Theory of Weight Control   **90**
Fallacies of Weight Control   **92**
Determining Percent of Calories from Fat   97
Chapter Summary   98

Closing Commentary   99
Fitness and Fallacies Self-Test   101
About the Authors   103

About the Meadow Brook Health Enhancement Institute

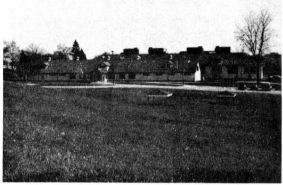

As a division of Oakland University, the institute's role and mission includes education and service to the southeastern Michigan community and research in disease prevention.

Meadow Brook Health Enhancement Institute staff members are people who have chosen to specialize in various areas of health promotion and disease prevention. Their fields of expertise include medicine, exercise physiology, medical technology, nutrition, cardiac rehabilitation, aerobics and recreational sports.

Oakland University faculty members and graduate students conduct research at the institute and many area physicians work with and contribute to institute programs.
Meadow Brook Health Enhancement Institute, Oakland University, Rochester, Michigan 48309-4401

CHAPTER 1

Exercise as
an Industry

Exercise is big business in the United States. Exercise publications, products, services and facilities are prevalent nationwide, and many Americans belong to health clubs, exercise studios and gyms. Millions of Americans perform aerobic exercise 100 or more days per year*. Statistics show that 10.3 million Americans perform fitness walking, 8.1 million run or jog, 4.9 million ride bicycles and 2.6 million swim. These and other exercise enthusiasts buy products and services from this multi-billion dollar industry. Unfortunately, much time and money are wasted on ineffective programs, products and services.

Competition for the exercise dollar has resulted in a variety of creative marketing programs, most of which promote the image of physical attractiveness that Americans value. While many benefits are obtained from regular physical exercise, the desire to improve appearance is probably the major force behind the start of many exercise programs, purchases of exercise-related products and the use of a variety of cosmetic exercise services.

The exercise industry, which includes health clubs, exercise studios, exercise salons, gyms and equipment shops, frequently has not employed competent personnel. While it often is assumed that employees of these facilities are well trained, many in fact have had little education in fields related to exercise. Unfortunately, many Americans have been guided in their exercise programs by individuals with little understanding of exercise physiology. Lack of training through recognized exercise organizations and the promotion of fallacies or unsafe practices represent areas of major concern.

Several nationally recognized organizations (i.e., The American College of Sports Medicine) have developed excellent training programs for exercise industry personnel. As a result, there has been an improvement in the expertise of some who lead exercise or advise the public in matters related to exercise.

Since no license is required to conduct an exercise-related business, training and certification of personnel are largely voluntary. Many individuals who regularly direct exercise programs lack basic familiarity with human anatomy, physiology,

* *U.S. News and World Report,* July 18, 1988 (page 54).

safety and emergency procedures. The exercise knowledge of many people who direct physical activity is derived, in part, form misleading information in fitness magazines and exercise video tapes and from fallacies passed from one person to another. The public is repeatedly presented with inaccurate or unsupported statements regarding matters of exercise. Such statements are made frequently for the purpose of selling a magazine, health club membership or fitness device. As exercise fallacies are repeated, they are frequently accepted as truths and then become traditions.

The print media, especially fitness magazines and "women's" magazines, often are major contributors to fallacies regarding body toning, one of the most misunderstood concepts of exercise. Magazines tend to print what sells best: headlines promising an attractive body with little effort tend to promote strong sales. Over the past few years popular magazines have offered the reader solutions to problems such as flabby thighs, unflattering waistlines, sagging fannies and soft upper arms. The prevalence of these articles has deceived millions.

The purpose of this book is to identify the myths associated with exercise and to present established principles which are important in the development of an exercise program. Particular emphasis has been placed on the design of an exercise program which is as time-efficient, safe and effective as possible. This guide provides a scientific perspective of exercise which promotes the development of desirable appearance as well as the improvement or maintenance of aerobic fitness, flexibility, muscular strength and muscular endurance. These concepts will be discussed in a manner consistent with established principles of exercise physiology.

CHAPTER 2

The Myth of Body Toning

Body toning is one of the most misunderstood concepts of exercise. Terminology frequently associated with toning includes muscle toning, inch loss, body sculpting, and body shaping. This concept is among the most heavily promoted misconceptions in exercise. The promotion involves the suggestion that undesirable body contours are due to poorly toned muscles and that these contours may be reshaped, sculpted or toned through regional exercise.

Americans assume that muscle tone enhances appearance: the more tone, the better the appearance. However, since no practical method exists to measure muscle tone, its assessment is very subjective. General appearance is often the criterion used to evaluate muscle tone. Unfortunately, this type of subjective evaluation may be a poor indicator of tone. Muscle tissue is covered by a layer of adipose tissue (fat) and skin, and the nature of these two types of tissue may affect appearance much more than muscle tone. While it is true that under certain conditions specific body regions may be reshaped through regional exercise, the degree to which this may be accomplished depends greatly on the body composition of the individual in question and the design of the exercise program employed. Body fat and loose skin cannot be reshaped through exercise.

Regional Exercise

Regional exercise consists of repetitious movements which affect specific areas of the body, such as the thighs, hips, abdomen and arms (especially the backs of the arms in women). Promotions for this kind of exercise suggest that if a particular region of the body is exercised, that region will become toned and more attractive. The terms tone or toned refer to a certain appearance which is characterized by a firm, lean body. In the design of regional exercise programs, very important principles of exercise physiology frequently are ignored. These principles will be discussed in this and proceeding chapters.

Spot Reduction

Spot reducing is a procedure which is speculated to cause the reduction of body fat from a specific area or areas of the body. This procedure employs specific regional exercises such as thigh and abdominal exercises for the purpose of preferentially removing fat from these areas. The misconception is that "saddlebag hips" can be reduced by repeated contractions of the abductor muscles of the outer thigh. Also promoted is the misconception that the abdominal "spare tire" may be reduced by repeated contractions of the abdominal muscles. The concept of spot reduction often is applied inappropriately to other problem areas of the body. Research has failed to demonstrate that spot reduction, regardless of the number of repetitions, can cause a decrease of fat in a particular body region. In practical terms, spot reduction is not possible.

The types of regional exercises employed for the purpose of spot reduction are among those which require the least caloric expenditure and therefore are unlikely to result in a caloric deficit and a significant fat loss. A basic principle of general weight reduction involves expending more calories than are consumed. A caloric deficit is then created, causing a reduction of body fat.

Even aerobic exercise which provides a meaningful caloric expenditure, such as brisk walking, jogging or bicycling, does not result in a greater loss of body fat from the exercised leg region as compared to other regions of the body. If spot reduction were possible, then the thousands of contractions of the leg muscles which take place in a one-hour walk or bicycle ride would cause more fat to be lost from the legs than from other areas. It is quite clear that such regional exercise does not cause fat to be lost preferentially from any part of the leg.

Aerobic exercise is, however, the type of activity which is more likely to result in a caloric deficit and weight loss because of its comparatively great caloric expenditure. During weight loss, body fat tends to be removed from all areas of the body or by a pattern of fat reduction which is determined hereditarily. We all have individual patterns of fat deposition and fat withdrawal which are not altered by exercise. If you hope to reduce a body region, you must first determine the potential for fat loss. If a significant amount of body fat exists in the region to be reduced, then an overall weight loss must be produced with the hope that body fat will be diminished in the desired area.

Shaping, Sculpting and Toning

In many exercise classes, especially dance-exercise classes, body shaping, sculpting or toning is an important part of the exercise hour. Many individuals who take part in exercise classes do so, at least in part, to improve problem areas of the body. Many women are unhappy with their thighs, hips or upper arms. Men frequently express concern with their waistlines. Most people hope that their exercise efforts will result in general toning and improved appearance. Often, the ultimate goal is to acquire a firm or "hard" body. After all, the right appearance brings social rewards. Getting rid of the "saddlebag hips" or "spare tire" is paramount.

With these goals in mind, participants frequently expect to be taken through a workout which focuses, at least in part, on these problem areas. The misconception is that thigh exercises will shape the thighs, that abdominal exercises will sculpt the abdomen and that upper arm exercises will tone flabby arms. Given the public interest in body shaping, exercise instructors try to accommodate clients' desires. Therefore, in many exercise classes, regional exercises are done in a group setting on the floor, with body weight, portions of body weight and light ankle or hand weights as resistance. Unfortunately this type of exercise program is rarely effective.

Summary of the Effect of Common Toning Exercises Performed on the Floor (With Little or No Equipment)

- No cardiovascular conditioning
- Very little caloric expenditure
- No effect on the resting metabolic rate
- No effect on the adipose (fat) mass
- Little or no effect on muscular strength
- Little or no effect on muscular endurance
- Even with adequate overload, appearance may be improved only when the adipose mass is small
- If benefits occur, much time is required
- No toning or shaping of skin or fat
- Improvement may be perceived when none has actually taken place (a misperception due to the expectation of improved appearance)

The leg lift shown in figure 2.1 is a common floor exercise and requires the contraction of the abductors (outer thigh muscles). When these muscles are worked with many repetitions, fatigue and a somewhat painful burning sensation may result. Frequently this burning sensation is used erroneously as evidence of a good regional workout; that is, exercise which will shape, sculpt or tone the outer thigh. The same principle is mistakenly applied to other body regions. However, the fatigue, and especially the burning sensation, are actually the result of inadequate oxygen supply to the muscle. "The burn" will be discussed more thoroughly in Chapter 3.

5

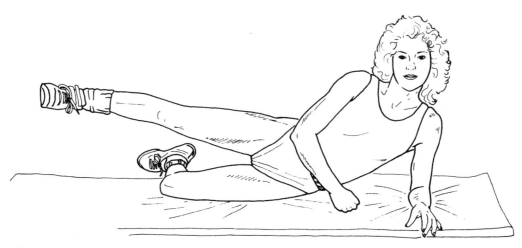

Figure 2.1 The outer thigh leg lift or lateral leg lift, even with the use of weights, represents a poor use of time.

As discrepancies between traditional exercise procedures and well-established principles of exercise physiology become more apparent, some interesting questions are asked.

    I. What is muscle tone?
        a. Do group exercises, done on the floor, improve muscle tone?
        b. Do group exercises, done on the floor, improve appearance?
        c. What type of tissue can be reshaped or toned?
    II. What is the cause of undesirable body contours?
    III. What is happening as a person becomes more visibly toned?
    IV. What is the most effective method to acquire the toned look?
    V. How can tone be objectively measured?

The examination and application of certain principles of exercise physiology may shed some light on these areas of question.

Muscle Tonus (Muscle Tone)

Muscle tonus is a term which refers specifically to muscle tissue. The definition of muscle tonus makes no reference to the appearance of a body region but only to specific characteristics of muscle tissue itself.

Herbert deVries, in his fourth edition of *Physiology of Exercise**, states that resting muscle tonus is the result of a state of partial contraction of muscle tissue

---

*deVries, Herbert A, *Physiology of Exercise,* Fourth edition, 1988, William C. Brown Publishers, College Division, Dubuque, Iowa.

caused in part by a more or less constant state of activity in a small portion of muscle fibers in a muscle. deVries goes on to state that, given current research, muscle tonus appears to have two components:

Active Component. The active component is the result of neural activity, that is, the firing of certain motor neurons which signal muscles to contract. At any given time when a muscle is at rest, only a small portion of the muscle fibers may be firing. Some research has indicated that under certain conditions, a resting muscle may become electrically silent for brief periods of time.

Passive Component. The passive component is the result of the elasticity of muscle and connective tissue plus the result of tissue turgor. Tissue turgor refers to the pressure of certain cellular and intracellular body fluids and the effect of this pressure on surrounding tissue. For example, immediately after a strenuous workout with weights or other resistance equipment, muscles may be a little larger and firmer. The person is said to be "pumped." This effect is the result of a temporary increase in tissue turgor. Much of this effect is lost within an hour following the training session.

The effects of exercise training on resting muscle tonus have not been clearly demonstrated in well-controlled research settings. Assumptions are based on empirical evidence (observation by trial and error). *However, a training program which is effective in the measurable improvement of muscular strength or muscular endurance is likely to be effective in the improvement of muscle tonus.* This is an important concept which will be discussed later.

From the preceding discussion of muscle tonus it should be clear that these concepts refer only to muscle tissue. There is no evidence that non-contractile tissue, such as fat or skin, may be toned through exercise training. Elasticity is evident in fat tissue and skin tissue, but it does not seem to be affected by exercise. Heredity and age may be greater factors related to the elasticity and appearance of these tissues.

Since only muscle tissue may be toned through exercise, it is important to be aware that when muscle tissue is covered by excess adipose tissue, improved muscle tone may not be visibly evident. Furthermore, improvement of muscle tone is likely to take place only when the exercise training includes adequate muscular overload. The concept of overload will be discussed in more detail shortly.

The Cause of Undesirable Body Contours

Millions of Americans are overfat. Surveys indicate that the number of pounds of fat per capita has been steadily increasing for many years. In this country, adults commonly gain one to three pounds of total body weight every year. In a 1984 lecture, Jack Wilmore, Ph.D., currently of the University of Texas at Austin, stated that between the ages of 25 and 55 the average American gains 30 pounds of total body weight. He suggests that this change of body composition is the net result of 45 pounds of additional fat and 15 pounds of reduced lean mass. This loss of lean mass comes mostly from muscle mass and bone mass.

The author has coined the term *adult atrophy* to describe this gradual change in body composition seen so frequently in American adults. The major cause of adult atrophy is insufficient physical activity. People who are insufficiently active don't stimulate muscles adequately to maintain the lean mass (muscle mass). As a result, the muscle mass gradually diminishes throughout adulthood. The upper body seems to demonstrate the greatest loss of muscular strength, muscular endurance and muscle mass. As muscle mass is lost, the resting metabolic rate declines. Muscle mass is more metabolically active than fat tissue, even at rest. As the muscle mass is reduced, the need for calories is also reduced. Daily resting metabolic rate is a significant variable in determining caloric expenditure. As resting metabolism decreases, appetite does not diminish equally and the result is a gradual increase in body fat. An important benefit of exercise is that these effects could be diminished or prevented with regular aerobic exercise, which could also help to maintain lean body mass.

It is clear that undesirable body contours are much more likely to be caused by excess body fat than by poor muscle tone. The authors have performed thousands of body composition evaluations and have yet to find one person with an undesirable abdominal, thigh or hip protrusion who did not have a large amount of fat in that region. "Saddle bag hips," "sagging fannies" and "spare tires" are not

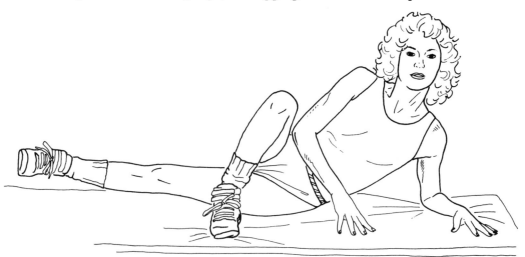

Figure 2.2 The inner thigh leg lift, even with the use of weights, is not likely to tone the inner thigh.

likely to be caused by hanging or protruding muscles. "Saddle bag hips," "sagging fannies" and "spare tires" are almost always caused by excess fat. When the regional fat is reduced as the result of an overall weight loss, these undesirable body contours will improve.

The thigh and hip regions are the least likely areas of the body to demonstrate a lack of muscle tonus, even in a non-exerciser. Even sedentary individuals use these muscles to move their body weight from one place to another. Normal daily activities are sufficient to maintain some muscle tonus in these regions. One reason that the strength of thigh and hip muscles is very comparable in men and women is that both men and women must carry their own weight. Upper body strength between the sexes, however, is generally quite different. (Although cultural gender differences regarding upper body activity are diminishing, females still tend to perform fewer activities which result in the development of upper body strength.) Therefore, since lower body muscle tonus usually is reasonably well-developed for both men and women, further improvements require a substantial degree of muscular overload. This kind of overload is likely to require the use of heavy weights or

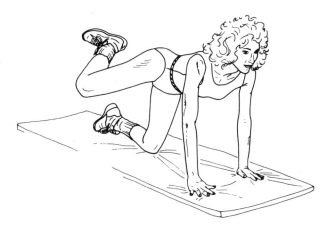

Figure 2.3 The "hydrant" is done to tone the outer thigh and hip regions. This concept is a common exercise fallacy.

other progressive resistance exercise equipment (Nautilus, Cybex, Paramount, Universal, etc.). Improvements in muscular strength and tonus are unlikely to result from the exercises shown in Figures 2.1, 2.2, 2.3 and 2.4. Recommendations for muscular strength and muscular endurance training are provided in Chapter 3.

It has been stated that the adductor muscles (inner thigh) and abductor muscles (outer thigh) get little use in normal activities and that because of this, the exercises shown in Figures 2.1 and 2.2 will provide effective training for these regions. This concept is clearly an exercise fallacy. Electromyography (study of the electrical ac-

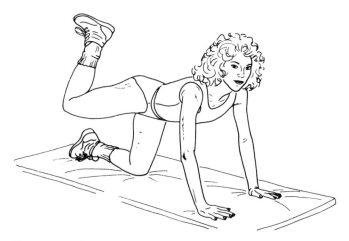

Figure 2.4 The donkey kick is also used to tone the thigh and hip regions. Other activities are more effective for the improvement of appearance and the development of muscular strength and endurance.

tivity of muscles) of the thigh region during walking, jogging and dance-exercise has revealed that all areas of the thigh are highly active. The adductors and abductors are important stabilizers of the thigh.

To demonstrate the work of the abductors, a simple procedure can be performed. First stand with weight evenly distributed on both feet. Place the right thumb 2–3 inches below the right iliac crest (top of the hip bone). The somewhat soft abductor muscles should be palpable. Next, while holding the right thumb in this position, shift the body weight to the right foot (Fig. 2.5). With this positional change, the tissue under the right thumb should suddenly become noticeably firmer as these muscles contract to stabilize the level of both iliac crests. Without the vigorous contraction of the abductor muscle group, the left iliac crest would fall. The contraction of these muscles is much more vigorous as the body weight is thrust upon each foot with every step in jogging and dance-exercise. The tension created by these muscles in normal daily activities is greater than the tension created in the exercises shown in Figure 2.1. Therefore there is little support for the inclusion of these leg lifts, including exercises known as ''hydrants,'' in an exercise session.

As evidence of adductor utilization in normal activities, anyone who has had a groin strain (adductor strain) can describe the pain created by walking. The acts of jogging or dance-exercise become excruciating when this muscle group is injured. A groin strain can disable athletes for weeks.

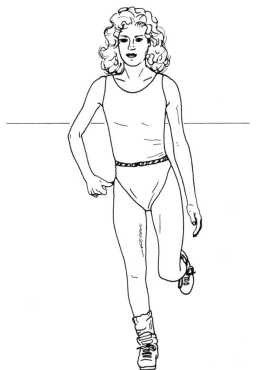

Figure 2.5 A demonstration of the use of the abductor (outer thigh) muscles during aerobic exercise.

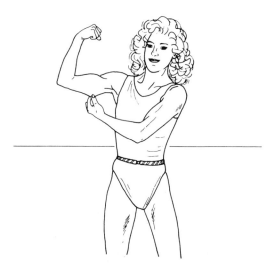

Figure 2.6 The determination of regional body composition. When muscles are voluntarily contracted, remaining loose tissue is untonable fat and skin.

If one wishes to improve the appearance of the thighs and hips, is there a reason to perform outer thigh, inner thigh or hip exercises, even with heavy weights? The answer is no, unless the individual is willing to put forth the kind of training effort demonstrated by body builders. These individuals may train with heavy weights for a total of 18 to 24 hours per week.

It has been argued that proper weight training of the inner thighs, outer thighs and hips will tend to improve the strength and endurance of these muscles, thus making this training worthwhile. However, the training of these areas is unlikely to result in an improved functionality. That is, it does not seem likely that this training would enhance movement or performance in a meaningful way.

The cause of undesirable body contours can be further investigated by an analysis of regional body composition. For example, if an individual has "flabby upper arms," one can determine whether the cause is excess body fat. If it is recognized that muscle tissue is contractile in nature and that fat tissue and skin tissue are not, then a method to analyze regional body composition should become apparent. To determine the composition of the "flabby" tissue of the triceps region, first make a fist, contracting *all* of the muscles of the arm. The muscles of the entire arm including the triceps region will be firm and taut. Remaining tissue which is soft to the touch and which may be pinched into a fold of tissue is either adipose or skin tissue. Remember, excess fat cannot be spot reduced or toned. Only muscle tissue can be toned. This analysis applies to any body region.

What Happens as a Person Becomes More Visibly Toned?

Countless people in a variety of exercise programs have been pleased with improvements in appearance. Many of these people have performed exercise which has included typical floor work employing light resistance and many repetitions. Others have done only aerobic exercise. Others have only changed eating habits. Many individuals have performed a combination of these strategies. Since people often have employed more than one strategy at a given time, it may have been difficult to determine which procedures were effective and which were not. Often, toning exercises done on the floor are given the credit when in fact they have been quite ineffective.

The appearance of improved tone is often the result of the loss of body fat as long as the amount of fat lost is not so great as to cause the skin to become flaccid. Aside from the problem of excess skin, moderate weight loss, even in the absence of exercise, may produce an appearance of improved tone. When body fat is reduced, the shape, size and tonus of muscles may be more obvious. Even in a non-exerciser, the existing nature of muscle may have a more pleasing appearance. A well-designed program of muscular strength and endurance further improves the appearance of the exercised areas as long as regional fat is minimal.

When someone has been overfat for a long time, the skin grows to accommodate body size. When a lot of fat is lost, excessive skin remains. Having limited elasticity, the skin may not conform well to the new body size. No exercise can correct flaccid skin. (Cosmetic surgery has been used with varying degrees of success to correct this problem.)

A few individuals, even after achieving recommended weight, may still have a region of the body which contains excess fat. This seems especially true of the hip and thigh regions of some women. The reduction of fat in these regions may be impractical, requiring a total percent of body fat which is well below the desirable range of 19% to 25%. At such a low percent of body fat, the thighs and hips may look acceptable, but the remainder of the body may appear emaciated or anorectic. Furthermore, the risk for a number of health disorders is increased.

An important concept which people, especially women, should accept is that few individuals can attain the standard of beauty held before us by the commercial media. Many individuals feel that failure to attain these standards of physical attractiveness represents a personal failure and poor self esteem often results. It is possible to improve appearance, but generally only within a certain range which is determined hereditarily. Most people with body contours considered to be attractive by our society were born with a predisposition to a specific body type. When

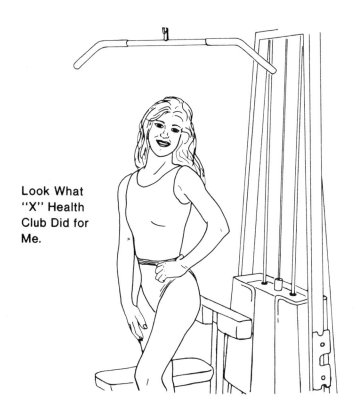

Look What
"X" Health
Club Did for
Me.

an attractive person advertises a sugar substitute, skin cream or health club, remember that it is extremely unlikely that the advertised product created the model's physical attractiveness. Some people simply have inherited the "right stuff."

Acquiring The Toned Look

The most effective means of acquiring the toned look involves the utilization of proper aerobic exercise, good nutritional habits and a well-designed program of muscular strength and muscular endurance. Details of these three components will be discussed in proceeding chapters.

How Can Tone be Measured Objectively?

If body composition goals are to be reached, it is essential to have an objective means to measure and evaluate progress. The problem with toning is that there is no objective, practical method to measure or evaluate progress. The concept of toning is very subjective. The elusiveness of the toning concept is exploited by those who market various body toning services. People who commit themselves economically and psychologically to a particular program tend to perceive improvement subjectively when none actually may have taken place. In all probability, the perception of improved tone associated with some forms of exercise is simply a placebo effect.

Conversely, aerobic capacity, nutritional habits and changes in muscular strength and muscular endurance may be objectively quantified. Through field or laboratory analyses, aerobic fitness may be analyzed. Through computer analysis of a seven-day nutritional diary, dietary patterns can be determined. Through field or laboratory analysis, muscular strength and muscular endurance may be compared to age group norms as well as to previous performance. In any of these areas, improvement can be clearly quantified. *When muscular strength and endurance are meaningfully improved, then muscle tone is likely to be improved.*

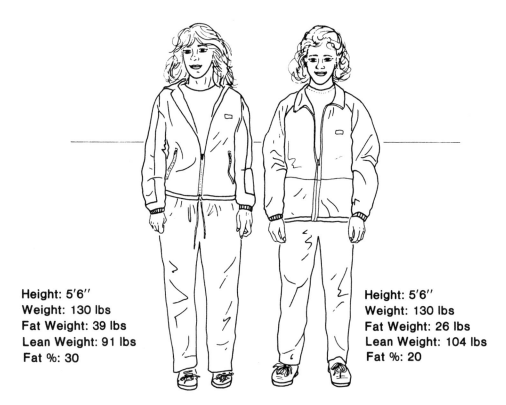

Height: 5'6"
Weight: 130 lbs
Fat Weight: 39 lbs
Lean Weight: 91 lbs
Fat %: 30

Height: 5'6"
Weight: 130 lbs
Fat Weight: 26 lbs
Lean Weight: 104 lbs
Fat %: 20

Figure 2.7 Body composition of two individuals having the same height, weight and gender.

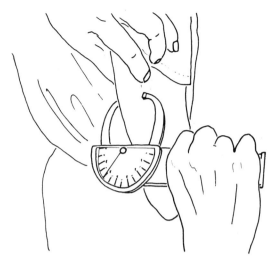

Figure 2.8 Skinfold Body Composition Analysis.

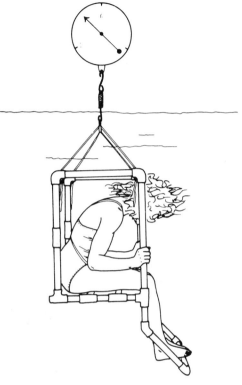

Figure 2.9 Hydrostatic Body Composition Analysis.

Body Composition

Since the amount of fat that the body carries has such a strong influence upon appearance, some basic concepts of body composition should be understood. First, total body weight is frequently a poor indicator of body composition. Changes in total body weight may correlate poorly with changes in the amount of body fat. Furthermore, height should not be used to determine desirable weight. Two individuals of the same sex, height and weight may have very different amounts of body fat. One individual may have more lean mass (i.e., muscle) and the other more fat.

It is important to understand that when an individual loses weight, the loss may come from body components other than fat. Lean mass and body fluids may be substantially reduced by a variety of weight loss procedures. Lean mass plus fat mass plus body fluids equal total body weight. Desirable weight loss should occur as the result of a reduction in body fat. Depending on a number of environmental and nutritional factors, the weight of body fluids may vary by two to ten pounds or more in one day. Therefore, the emphasis of a weight control program should be placed on the reduction of excess body fat.

Hydrostatic weighing (underwater weighing) is among the most accurate procedures available for determining body composition and recommended weight. Skinfold analysis is reasonably accurate when performed by a technician with considerable experience and who has had many opportunities to compare skinfold analysis to hydrostatic weighing of the same subject.

Hydrostatic weighing is based on the principle that, in water, muscle sinks and fat floats. The heavier an individual is underwater, as compared to his or her dry land weight, the leaner the individual is. As body fat is reduced (and muscle mass remains constant), underwater weight should increase.

Body composition procedures which are not recommended include impedance analysis and any procedure which attempts to quantify total body fat through measurement of only one site on the body. At this time impedance analysis has not been found to be an accurate indicator of body fat percent over a wide range of body types. The impedance instrument measures the amount of body water present at a given time. Lean tissue and fat tissue contain remarkably different amounts of water. Muscle contains significantly more water than fat. Currently, converting the amount of body water to an estimate of body fat is not considered sufficiently accurate. Many factors can influence the amount of fluid present in the human body at a given time. Given a choice of hydrostatic weighing, skinfold analysis and impedance analysis, the preferred choice would be hydrostatic weighing followed by skinfold analysis. Some formulas which utilize circumference measurements are reasonably accurate for certain groups.

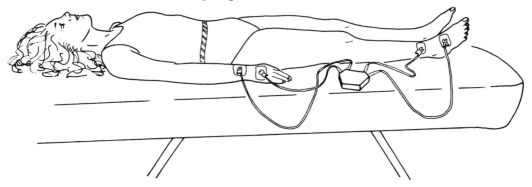

Figure 2.10 Electrical Impedance Body Composition Analysis.
Some researchers who have tested this equipment do not recommend it.

The recommended percents of body fat provided by the Meadow Brook Health Enhancement Institute at Oakland University, Rochester, Michigan, are as follows:

Body Composition Recommendations

	Athletes	*Others*
Men	not less than 5%	9% – 15%
Women	not less than 12%	19% – 25%

Notice that recommended percents do not change with age. While body fat may increase with age in the United States, there is no physiological reason that this *should* happen. For those who experience a decrease in lean body weight (muscle) with age, total weight should *decrease* with age. This is contrary to the commonly held clinical belief that, because Americans frequently become heavier and fatter as they get older, this change in body composition is acceptable.

Toning Tables and Electronic Muscle Stimulation

One of the hottest new exercise businesses, fraught with deception and misconception, involves body toning through passive exercise. Body toning salons which appear under a number of nameplates offer sweatless, effortless exercise which is guaranteed to provide inch loss though not necessarily weight loss. For the entrepreneur, start-up costs are comparatively minimal requiring the rental of a store front and purchase of equipment. Given the attractiveness of the claims and the number of people who want to exercise in the supine position, the investment is often returned quickly. Neither the government nor the public has required the operators of these businesses to be credentialed or to demonstrate the effectiveness of their claims. As a result, almost anyone can operate this type of business.

Two methods of passive exercise are currently in use. One employs toning tables, also called toning beds, on which participants do little more than lie down. The tables are designed to move the body with the use of an electric motor. Six or seven different tables are used in series for 10 minutes each. The sit-up table (Fig 2.11) is designed with a hinge in the center. While the participant lies on the table, the device raises and lowers the torso in a sit-up fashion. Entrepreneurs claim that ten minutes on this table is equivalent to 90 or more sit-ups. The physiology involved with this movement does not support this claim. The leg table (Fig 2.12) has elevated boots similar to those found on water skis. As the feet are held above the level of the torso, the legs are moved in a circular motion. Claims have been made that this movement tones the legs, slims the thighs, firms the hips and is equivalent to a two-mile walk. This result is very unlikely. This form of exercise is passive and, therefore, heart rate remains at or very near resting levels. This machine cannot possibly simulate a two-mile walk. Even world class racewalkers are unable to walk two miles in ten minutes. Only highly conditioned runners are capable of completing two miles in ten minutes. Covering two miles in ten minutes is not even remotely similar, physiologically, to lying on a leg table for ten minutes. Well-established principles of exercise physiology indicate that this system cannot improve fitness, cannot make fat go away and is unlikely to tone muscles. The claims associated with these toning tables represent one of the most outrageous consumer frauds in the United States today.

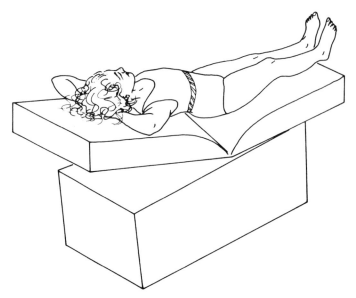

Figure 2.11 Sit-up Table (Passive Exercise).

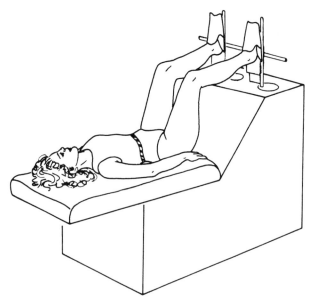

Figure 2.12 Leg Table (Passive Exercise).

Many exercise entrepreneurs appear to be caring, sincere people. However, most lack sufficient educational background in exercise physiology to operate competently. One entrepreneur was quoted as saying that these tables help to "break down fat." Furthermore, it was suggested that if the participant drinks six to eight glasses of water each day, the fat which is broken down will be flushed from the body in the urine. The statement was made in the belief that it was accurate. Unfortunately, this claim is nothing short of malpractice. The fraudulent claims made by this entrepreneur have been made by many other operators of fitness and weight loss businesses.

It seems inappropriate that while hair dressers must pass state board exams, anyone can operate an exercise, nutrition or weight control business and misinform the public in a manner which may detrimentally influence health.

Another method of passive exercise receiving much attention is electronic muscle stimulation. This procedure also requires the participant to lie on a table. Electrodes are attached to the area of the body to be stimulated and the current is turned on. A tingling sensation is felt as muscles contract. The current may be increased to cause more vigorous contractions but, for most, the sensation caused by strong electrical current is too painful. Regardless of the amount of current used,

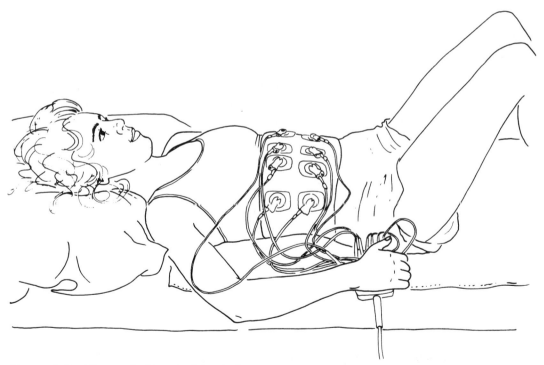

Figure 2.13 Electronic Muscle Stimulation.

when the electrodes are attached to the abdominal region, the contractions are very unlikely to approach the intensity of one sit-up. The muscles contract but they do not shorten. A common claim is that a 30-minute session with electrodes attached to the abdomen is equivalent to over one thousand sit-ups. Claims of effortless "inch loss" are also made. As has already been discussed, abdominal protrusions are due to excess body fat. Even one thousand sit-ups performed every day would not have a meaningful effect on abdominal fat. Furthermore, if one-thousand sit-ups were performed in 30 minutes, heart rate and breathing rate would change dramatically. While on the table, little, if any, physiological change occurs. This observation provides sufficient evidence that electronic muscle stimulation has little effect on the muscles of an apparently healthy, normal individual. Electronic muscle stimulation and mechanical tables do have a meaningful purpose in the field of physical therapy but provide no benefit in body toning or fitness of the able-bodied.

The Fallacy of Body Toning: A Typical Scenario

Each of us has body areas which we would like to firm and trim. Therefore, many people do toning exercises. Only muscle can be toned, fat cannot. Do you really lack muscle tone or do you have too much fat? This may be determined with a simple test.

> The upper arm can be used as an example to determine whether or not loose tissue is fat or muscle. Hold your arm parallel to the floor and make a tight fist, contracting all the muscles of the arm. When muscle is contracted, it is firm and taut. All tissue which remains soft is either fat or skin.

If you have a considerable amount of fat or loose skin, toning exercises will not "firm up those soft spots." Toning exercises cannot tone or reduce fat or skin. This test can be applied to any body region.

Most undesirable body contours are due to excess body fat. The type of exercise most likely to reduce excess body fat is aerobic exercise. Aerobic exercise results in a greater caloric expenditure than other types of exercise and is the form of activity most likely to reduce body fat. Unfortunately, the pattern of fat loss you experience is hereditary. There is no exercise which causes fat to be lost from a preferred area.

Chapter Summary

- Body toning is a vague and misunderstood concept.
- Regional exercise cannot reduce or reshape body fat or skin.

- Only well-designed programs of regional exercise which utilize adequate overload are likely to reshape or tone.
- In the presence of excess fat, well-toned muscles may not be apparent.
- Regional exercise requires less caloric expenditure than aerobic exercise.
- Everyone has a genetically determined pattern of fat loss and fat deposition which is not altered by exercise.
- Aerobic exercise is more effective in the reduction of body fat than regional exercise.
- Many individuals are motivated to join exercise classes by the social rewards of an enhanced physical appearance.
- It can be assumed that an exercise program which measurably improves muscular strength and endurance is necessary to improve muscle tone.
- "The burn" is caused by inadequate oxygen supply to skeletal muscles.
- Most undesirable body contours are due to excess body fat rather than poorly-toned muscles.
- The reduction of body fat alone may give the appearance of improved tone.
- Muscle tonus has two components: the active component and the passive component.
- Adult atrophy involves the reduction of the lean mass, the enlargement of the fat mass, and the reduction of functionality throughout adulthood.
- The cause of adult atrophy is insufficient physical activity.
- Flabby arms, abdomens, hips and thighs are not likely to become toned through regional exercise.
- Generally speaking, there is no need to perform exercises limited to the outer or inner thigh.
- Studies of electromyography indicate, though contrary to common claims, that inner and outer thigh muscles are quite active in normal aerobic activities.
- The thigh and hip regions are the least likely to demonstrate lack of muscle tonus.
- A simple procedure permits an analysis of regional body composition to distinguish between fat tissue and muscle tissue.
- Extreme physical attractiveness is often a genetic gift, rarely created through diet and exercise.

CHAPTER 3

Exercise, Fitness and "Looking Good"

Getting the Most with a Limited Amount of Time

Exercise is an important component of a lifestyle which is conductive to a high quality of life. Benefits of exercise include those listed in Table 3.1. Few individuals have an unlimited amount of time in which to exercise. Therefore, it is frequently desirable to design a exercise program which provides the greatest benefit in the time which one is willing to spend. The benefits of exercise may be classified into three categories: improved functionality, improved appearance and improved psychological state. Some benefits may be placed in more than one category. This chapter will deal primarily with the improvement of functionality with references to improved appearance.

Table 3.1
The Benefits of Regular Exercise

The following benefits are commonly-reported general effects of regular aerobic exercise performed according to recommendations made in this book.

- Improved appearance, muscle tone and posture
- Improved sense of well-being, self-image and self-confidence
- Reduced incidence or severity of psychological depression
- Reduction of the stress response
- Improved sleep patterns
- Reduction of restlessness and boredom
- Improved sense of energy

- Attainment and maintenance of a high level of functionality throughout life
- Reduction of body fat mass
- Augmentation of the lean body mass, especially in men.
- Maintenance of a higher resting caloric expenditure as compared to other methods of weight loss
- Increased caloric expenditure which facilitates weight loss
- Reduction of hunger

- Reduction of the set point (theoretical amount of body fat that the body automatically tends to store)
- Improved fat metabolism
- Improved management of diabetes (blood sugar)
- Maintenance of bone density with weight-bearing exercise
- Reduced incidence of constipation
- Improved heart function and circulation
- Improved ability to cope with warm, humid weather
- Improved resistance to cold environments
- Reduced incidence of muscle strains and other injuries which may occur in normal daily activities
- Reduction of blood fats such as triglyceride and LDL cholesterol
- Improvement of blood HDL cholesterol
- Reduction of blood pressure in hypertensive individuals
- Reduced risk of coronary artery disease and stroke

It is commonly assumed that as people grow older, they become less functional. Loss of functionality is frequently attributed exclusively to the aging process. Actually, most of the loss of physical working capacity seen in this country is not due to the aging process, but to a progressive pattern of long-term inactivity. The "use it or lose it" principle certainly applies to this concept. Many individuals who have remained adequately active throughout adulthood have lost very little or their

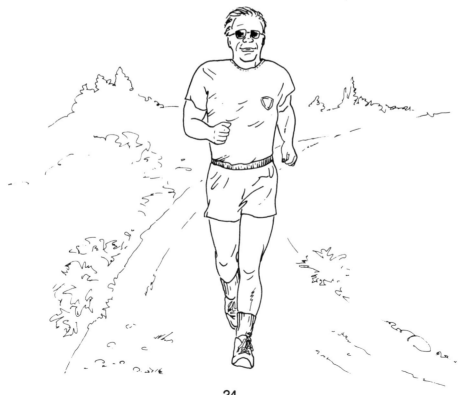

physical abilities. Some people in their sixties and beyond perform activities such as running, race walking, cycling, swimming and cross-country skiing, at levels well beyond those of more sedentary individuals in their twenties and thirties. This kind of functionality is the result of a commitment to a well-designed program of fitness. Certainly, aging is inevitable, but for many Americans it has been accentuated by inactivity.

In the design of an exercise program, four components should be considered.

Components of Fitness

Muscular Endurance
Muscular Strength
Cardiovascular Endurance (aerobic capacity)
Flexibility

It is generally recognized that cardiovascular endurance is the most important of the four fitness components since it has the greatest potential to influence overall health and functionality. However, to continue the discussion of muscle tone, muscular endurance and muscular strength will be discussed first.

Muscular endurance may be described as the ability to perform a submaximal task many times in succession. Muscular endurance may be evaluated by a number of methods. The endurance of certain upper body muscles can be measured by determining the number of push-ups or sit-ups which can be done consecutively. The ability to perform 30 push-ups is a demonstration of good muscular endurance of the pectoral and arm regions. Many people have the misconception that the ability to perform many push-ups is an indication of strength, rather than endurance. However, the inability to perform one push-up would suggest a strength limitation.

Muscular strength is best evaluated by determining the maximal amount of weight which can be lifted or moved one time. The strength of certain upper body muscles may be analyzed by determining the amount of weight which can be moved in the completion of one bench press (Fig. 3.2). The ability to bench press the equivalent of an individual's body weight represents good strength in men. For women, the ability to bench press 75% of an individual's weight represents good strength.

The Development of Muscular Strength, Muscular Endurance, Muscle Size and Muscle Tone

In the design of any exercise program, two important principles of exercise training should be recognized. One, *the overload principle,* frequently is not applied to exercise programs. In order to bring about a change in the characteristic of muscle, in

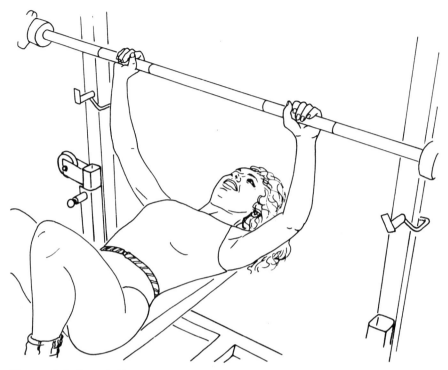

Figure 3.2 Bench Press.

either improved function or appearance, the muscle must create a tension or force near that of its maximal capacity to contract. In other words, the muscle must be provided with a workload that is well beyond normal daily activity. *The use of light resistance with many repetitions is much less productive.* An application of the overload principle can be made as follows: If in a program of muscular strength and endurance, the tension or force created by the muscle is so minimal that more than twenty-five repetitions can be performed, then the overload is inadequate.

With this principle in mind, the use of one-pound to three-pound ankle or hand weights is inadequate for most people to demonstrate an improvement in muscular strength, muscular endurance or muscle tone.

Equally important in the design of a muscular strength, endurance and toning program, is the *principle of progressive resistance.* This concept suggests that as the ability to increase the number of repetitions occurs over time, the resistance (weight) should be increased. Therefore, as ability improves, resistance should progress until goals of muscular strength, endurance or appearance are achieved.

As a general guideline for a program of muscular strength, endurance and toning, a weight should be selected which permits ten to fifteen repetitions. When a

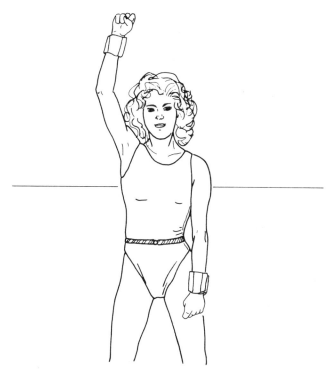

Figure 3.3 For the development of muscular strength, muscular endurance and toning, ankle and hand weights don't provide enough overload for most people.

greater number of repetitions can be performed, the resistance or weight should be increased.

Most modes of aerobic exercise provide training for the lower body only. Therefore, the upper body is frequently neglected, resulting in a gradual loss of upper body strength and muscle mass. The upper body should be emphasized in a fitness program of weight lifting.

The Program

The following suggestions for a program of progressive resistance exercise should provide meaningful results in a duration of approximately 30 minutes per day. The frequency of resistance exercise should be three times per week and the intensity or resistance should be determined by the weight which permits ten to fifteen repetitions. When more repetitions are possible, the resistance (weight) should be increased. For the first week or two, only one set of each exercise should be per-

27

formed to prevent soreness and muscle strains. Over the course of approximately one month, the number of sets (of 10 to 15 repetitions) of each exercise should increase from one to three. The first set should be done with lighter weight to permit a full fifteen repetitions. The initial set serves as a warm-up for each muscle group. When second and third sets are added, heavier weight may be used. For the last set, a weight should be used which permits only one to five repetitions. This kind of overload promotes more rapid development of strength and is recommended after about one month of resistance exercise.

Table 3.4
Summary of a Resistance Training Program

Set 1	Weight selection should permit fifteen repetitions.
Set 2	Added after one or two weeks, weight selection should permit only ten repetitions.
Set 3	Weight selection should permit only ten repetitions or
Set 3	Weight selection should permit only one to five repetitions. (This option should be included after one month of regular weight lifting.)

Safety should be of primary concern in establishing a weight lifting program. Good instruction in the proper set-up and use of equipment is essential. A capable spotter, such as an exercise partner, should be a prerequisite to the use of free weights.

Another safety concern when performing exercise for the development of muscular strength and muscular endurance involves breathing. It is not uncommon, when lifting weights or doing exercises such as push-ups or sit-ups, to perform a *valsalva maneuver*. A valsalva maneuver is performed by holding a breath, closing the glottis (structure which closes the windpipe) and forcefully exerting against the closed glottis as if to attempt to exhale. Sometimes a vocalization in the form of a quiet or loud grunt is made. The valsalva maneuver can cause the intrathoracic pressure (pressure in the chest cavity) to rise markedly, reducing the flow of blood from the lungs back to the heart, resulting in a decrease of cardiac (heart) output. This reduction of cardiac output may reduce the oxygen available to sensitive organs such as the heart and brain. Lightheadedness, spots or flecks of light before the eyes, and irregular heart rhythm may result. Systolic blood pressure may rise momentarily, well above 300 mmHg, during a valsalva maneuver. Normal resting values should be less than 140 mmHg. Systolic blood pressure during vigorous aerobic exercise should rise only to 160 to 190 mmHg. Frequent valsalva maneuvers may enlarge the right side of the heart. The valsalva maneuver should be avoided by exhaling on the exertion of a lift and inhaling on the recovery. In addition, breathing should not be interrupted.

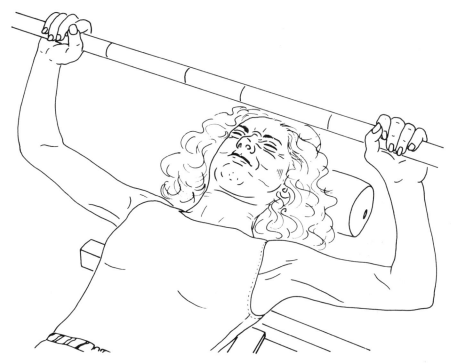

Figure 3.5 The Valsalva Maneuver

Recommended Resistance Exercise

(Note that exercises are arranged in pairs to work opposing muscle groups, though they may be completed in any order.)

Exercise	Major Muscle Groups
1. Chest Press (Fig. 3.6)	Pectorals, Triceps, Anterior Deltoids
2. Rowing Pull (Fig. 3.7)	Rhomboid, Latissimus Dorsi, Biceps
3. Shoulder Press (Fig.3.8)	Deltoids, Triceps
4. Lat Pull (Fig. 3.9)	Latissimus Dorsi, Biceps
5. Abdominal Crunch (Fig. 3.10)	Rectus Abdominus and other abdominal muscles
6. Back Extension (Fig. 3.11)	Erector Spinae group and Gluteal group

7. Leg Extension (Fig. 3.12)   Quadriceps

8. Leg Curl (Fig. 3.13)   Hamstrings

Exercises seven and eight are listed as optional for those who wish to enhance the lower body conditioning beyond the training provided by lower body aerobic exercise. For those who perform upper body aerobic exercise such a long-distance crawl stroke swimming, more attention should be given to the lower body.

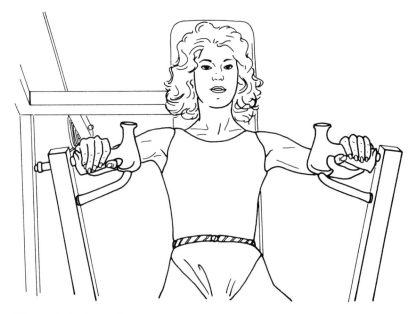

Figure 3.6 Chest Press

Misconceptions of Muscular Hypertrophy

Another important concept which is frequently misunderstood involves muscle enlargement or hypertrophy. Many women are concerned that if they lift heavier weights, they will develop large muscles. Muscular hypertrophy is perceived by some women to be undesirable and unattractive. The anabolic (muscular developing) properties of the male hormone testosterone result in muscular hypertrophy. The blood value of testosterone in females is about 10% of the amount found in males. *Because of lower testosterone values, it is unlikely that a woman would develop measurable muscular hypertrophy as the result of three weekly training*

30

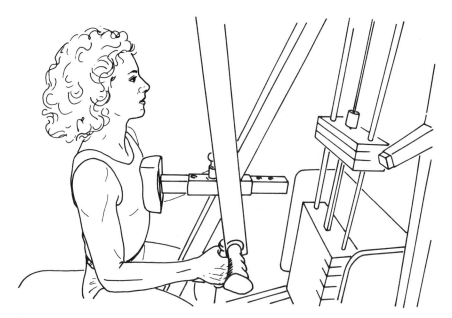

Figure 3.7 Rowing Pull

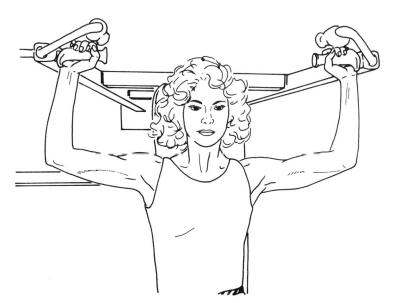

Figure 3.8 Shoulder Press

31

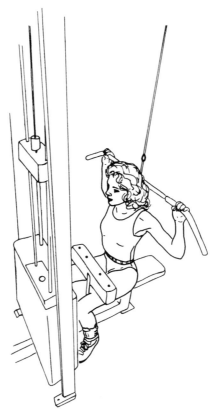

Figure 3.9 Lat Pull

sessions of 30 minutes to one hour, regardless of the weight used. The use of heavier weights would be more likely to improve the shape and tone of the muscles, however, the explanation of this phenomenon is not clearly understood. It is important to note that due to the lack of strength development, women generally have a greater potential than men to improve strength.

In a well-designed program of muscular strength and endurance, both men and women are likely to improve strength, but only men are likely to noticeably improve muscle size. Even for men, the development of noticeable hypertrophy is likely to require more than three sessions of thirty minutes per week, regardless of the amount of weight used. Many men experience difficulty when attempting to develop muscle size. Body type, an inherited characteristic, is a major factor which influences the ability to develop muscular hypertrophy. Ectomorphic (thin) men will experience more difficulty than mesomorphic (muscular) men.

Keep in mind that only muscle can be shaped or toned; fat and skin cannot. Therefore, even with regular weight lifting, a ''flabby'' region may not

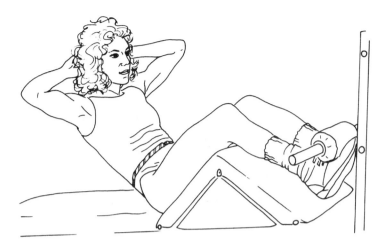

Figure 3.10 Abdominal Crunch (Spinal Flexion)

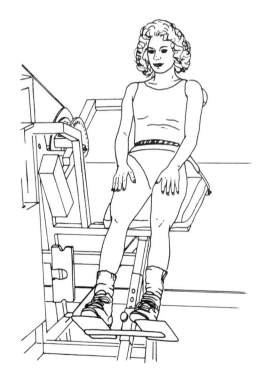

Figure 3.11 Back Extension

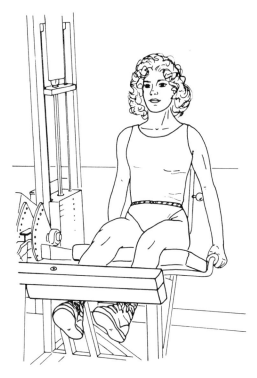

Figure 3.12 Leg Extension

demonstrate improved appearance until the fat is reduced. Aerobic exercise is the most appropriate activity to reduce body fat.

Questions have arisen about female body builders, the development of their bodies and the apparent contradictions to the concepts described above. The following observations may provide an explanation for the appearance of these women.

- Female body builders seen on television or in magazines have very unusual hereditary body characteristics and do not represent typical females. Most successful female body builders are genetically muscular. The typical female is as likely to become highly muscular through weight lifting as she is to become a marathon champion through jogging.

- Despite the body contours of female body builders, the ability to develop muscular hypertrophy is much more limited than in men. Female body builders have heights and weights which are very comparable to typical females. Male body builders are much more massive than typical males. Compared to male body builders, female body builders are much less muscularly massive.

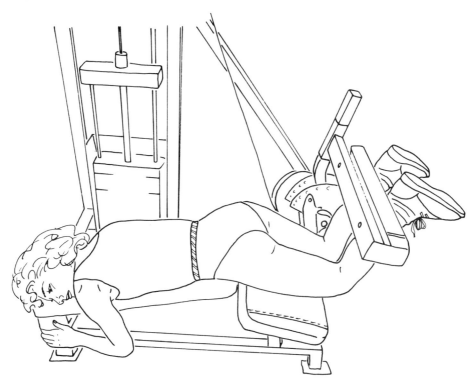

Figure 3.13 Leg Curl

- Female body builders are extremely lean, frequently having less that 10% bodyfat. Because female body builders have a much lower body fat content than typical female, muscles become more noticeable and better defined.
- The combination of tanned, oiled skin, the well-developed art of posing or displaying muscle groups and leanness results in an image of muscularity which otherwise would not be as apparent. Many muscular women who are not lean fail to have a muscular appearance because of superficial fat which lies between the skin and muscle. Fat tends to hide muscles.
- Female (and male) body builders may spend 18 to 24 hours or more per week involved in strenuous training. This time commitment represents far more training than the average female is likely to perform.
- The most competitive female body builders take every opportunity to win, sometimes at the risk of long-term health. The use of anabolic drugs (steroids) is quite common.

It should be clear that in terms of muscular strength, muscular endurance and appearance, women as well as men have much to gain through a well-designed program of progressive resistance exercise (weight lifting).

The Physiology of "The Burn"

Many exercisers assume that the painful burning sensation which follows a number of muscular repetitions is associated with extraordinary conditioning benefits, especially in terms of toning. It is also thought that exercises which don't generate "the burn" are less beneficial in this regard. Figures 2.1 and 2.3 are examples of calisthenic floor exercises frequently used to generate "the burn." In several exercise videotapes, well-known celebrities say "Now feel the burn!" While the fallacy of this concept is becoming well known by many exercise leaders, some clarification may be helpful.

To understand the physiology of "the burn," an understanding of aerobic metabolism and anaerobic metabolism is required.

Aerobic Metabolism. Aerobic metabolism occurs predominantly when work intensity is sufficiently low that adequate quantities of oxygen can be delivered to the exercising muscles at the time of need.

Anaerobic Metabolism. Anaerobic metabolism is achieved when physical activity is sufficiently intense that adequate quantities of oxygen cannot be delivered to the working skeletal muscles at the time of need.

Aerobic exercise may be described as physical activity which is moderate in intensity, rhythmic in nature, requires the use of large muscle groups and is completely continuous. The cardiovascular response to aerobic exercise is substantial, resulting in a cardiac (heart) output three to five times the resting rate.

Regional exercises, such as those shown in Figures 2.1 and 2.3, require the utilization of a comparatively small muscle mass. An important concept to understand regarding regional exercise is that the general cardiovascular response may be quite minimal. As a result, the blood flow to the working muscles may be considerably less than the blood flow to the same muscles during aerobic exercise which utilizes a much greater muscle mass. When doing lateral leg lifts, only the abductors are utilized. In lower-body aerobic exercise such as dance exercise and jogging, every skeletal muscle group below the waist is actively involved.

Since the cardiovascular response to regional exercise is limited, the oxygen supply will also tend to be quite limited. When muscles don't receive adequate oxygen at the time of need, anaerobic metabolism results. Skeletal muscles are capable of producing energy without adequate oxygen. However, there is a debt which the body must repay. During the production of energy without adequate oxygen (anaerobic metabolism), there is an accumulation of a substance known as lactic acid in the muscle tissue. Therefore lactic acid is a by-product of anaerobic metabolism. The accumulation of lactic acid causes, in part, the acute pain known as "the burn." When the activity is stopped, the lactic acid is removed by the circulation and "the burn" subsides. (It should be noted that lactic acid is not a waste product. Lactic acid is derived from glucose fuel [blood sugar] and may be converted back to glucose and used to produce energy at a later time.) The accumulation of lactic acid provides no toning benefits, and therefore "the burn" provides no advantage. The burning sensation only creates pain and a negative exercise experience.

On the other hand, the same abductor muscles used in Fig. 2.1 and 2.3 are part of the large muscle mass used in dance-exercise or jogging. There is a much greater blood flow and oxygen supply to those abductor muscles created by the accelerated cardiovascular response seen in aerobic exercise. The abductors are able to produce energy aerobically and therefore don't generate the accumulation of lactic acid in this form of exercise. The abductors may be performing more metabolic work for a much longer period of time but may not be creating "the burn."

Remember that "the burn" is merely evidence of anaerobic metabolism. It will result from something as simple as holding the arm extended from the shoulder for as little as two minutes. "The burn," by itself, does not necessarily mean that special benefit is occurring.

Cardiovascular Endurance: Aerobic Capacity

Individuals such as Joan Benoit-Samuelson and Bill Rodgers are well-known, world-class endurance athletes capable of extraordinary aerobic performance. These people have demonstrated the ability to run great distances at a pace of roughly five minutes per mile. Few people can run even one mile in the five-minute range. What makes Joan Benoit-Samuelson and Bill Rodgers different is their great capacity to metabolize (utilize) oxygen. The term *aerobic capacity* refers to the ability to use large amounts of oxygen. The more oxygen that can be delivered to working muscles and used to produce ATP (energy in the form of a substance known as adenosine triphosphate), the greater the aerobic performance will be. Two major factors influence this capacity:

1. Heredity
2. Training

Unfortunately, no matter how hard many individuals train, they will never acquire the metabolic abilities of the individuals mentioned above. The genetic predisposition of a high aerobic capacity must come first and then be developed through training.

Although most of us do not have the potential to develop world class athletic ability, there remain many important benefits associated with regular aerobic exercise (Table 3.1).

Since improved aerobic functioning is a result of aerobic exercise, virtually everyone can benefit from a well-designed program. The major mechanisms by which aerobic capacity improves include the following:

I. Improved cardiac (heart) function and improved ability to deliver oxygen to working muscles.

II. Improved ability of the muscle cells to metabolize delivered oxygen.

It should be noted that improved breathing is not listed among these most important mechanisms. Why, then, do sedentary individuals feel winded after climbing a few flights of stairs? The reason is associated with both the heart's ability to deliver oxygen and the muscle's ability to make energy *aerobically*. In the sedentary individual both mechanisms are compromised. As a result, metabolic by-products such as carbon dioxide are not removed efficiently by the circulation and eliminated by the lungs. Since carbon dioxide is a powerful stimulator of breathing, a sense of inadequate ventilation will be experienced.

Because of the enhanced cardiovascular ability of the regular aerobic exerciser, carbon dioxide is more efficiently eliminated and the urge to move large volumes of air is reduced. The trained individual may actually move less air per minute to do the same amount of work because of greater cardiovascular efficiency. *However, the amount of oxygen metabolized to do a given amount of work remains constant, regardless of the level of fitness.* The fit individual is capable of delivering the oxygen with fewer heartbeats (greater efficiency) and is capable of working at higher levels of oxygen utilization (greater aerobic capacity and performance).

Aerobic Exercise Prescription

A session of aerobic exercise should have three distinct components:

I. Warm-up
II. Aerobic Exercise
III. Cool Down

I. Warm-up

The primary emphasis of the warm-up should be to gradually increase heart rate in preparation for aerobic exercise. This initial period should warm the body and result in an increase in the core temperature. Some individuals, under certain environmental conditions, may begin to perspire by the end of the warm-up.

There is a great difference between the resting metabolic rate and the metabolic rate during aerobic exercise. The energy requirement of the resting metabolism is referred to as *one MET*. The MET is a metabolic unit used to quantify work relative to the resting metabolism. The metabolic rate during aerobic exercise may vary from 5–20 METs depending on the individual and the activity involved. Some cardiac or respiratory patients may be limited to 5 METs of activity while endurance athletes may be capable of performing 20 METs of work. The average person may perform aerobic exercise at 8–12 METs or an energy equivalent of 8–12 times the resting metabolic rate. The difference between one MET and 12 METs of exercise represents the magnitude of adjustment that the cardiovascular system must achieve every time aerobic exercise is performed by the healthy individual.

Without a gradual metabolic rise during aerobic exercise, the cardiovascular system may be inappropriately stressed. As a result, an irregular heart rhythm may take place. In some individuals, there may be a temporary lack of blood flow and oxygen to the muscle cells of the heart. Therefore, an initial cardiovascular adjustment period (warm-up) prior to an aerobic session is highly desirable.

The recommendations for warm-up are simple. First, warm-up should include the kind of activity to be performed during aerobic exercise. Second, the activity should begin very slowly and progress to the prescribed intensity over the course of 3 to 4 minutes.

II. Aerobic Exercise

There are four components of a prescription for aerobic exercise:

    a. Mode of activity
    b. Duration of activity
    c. Frequency of activity
    d. Intensity of activity

Mode

As described previously in this chapter, the activity performed during aerobic exercise should be completely continuous and rhythmic and should involve the large muscle groups of the body. Appropriate aerobic activities include walking, jogging, dance-exercise, swimming, cycling, rowing and cross-country skiing. The mode of activity most desirable for aerobic conditioning produces a fairly consistent intensity throughout the activity.

Court sports such as tennis, racquetball and basketball tend to be discontinuous and are less desirable. Preference should be given to achieving a high level of conditioning prior to participation in court sports. The intensity of exercise is difficult to control in these activities. With variations in intensity ranging from waiting for a serve to maximal exertion, court sports do not represent the ideal forms of activity for initial aerobic conditioning. However, after adequate aerobic conditioning has been achieved, high levels of aerobic capacity can be maintained by participating in court sports.

For many people, the best mode of aerobic exercise is brisk walking. Walking is an activity which most people can enjoy. Walking does not require special facilities or equipment. A good pair of walking or jogging shoes is all that is necessary. Walking is a gentle activity with a low incidence of exercise-induced injury. It permits the development and maintenance of a high level of fitness when performed according to the recommended duration, frequency and intensity.

Walking is not necessarily the preferred exercise for everyone. Personal preference in the selection of an activity is an important consideration. Other aerobic activities can be equally safe and beneficial. Performance of more than one mode of activity to provide variety is preferred by many people.

If aerobic exercise is to become a life-long commitment, it is essential that it be meaningful and enjoyable. For too many, exercise becomes a negative experience as people try to get into shape too quickly. As a result, people may quit the exercise program. To have an impact on the quality of life and a sense of well-being, aerobic exercise should become a habit to be maintained and enjoyed for a lifetime.

Duration

The recommended duration of aerobic exercise depends upon the mode of activity and the goals established for the program. Exercises which are more gentle to the musculo-skeletal system, such as walking swimming, cross country skiing, rowing and bicycling, may be performed for longer periods because over-use injuries are less likely to occur.

Because of the impact nature of jogging and dance-exercise (the foot striking the road or floor), these activities may require a more gradual progression of duration in order to reduce the risk of injury. For individuals with orthopedic or structural limitations, the duration of high-impact activities may have to be modified to prevent an exercise-related injury.

If, in addition to improved aerobic capacity, goals include a reduction of body fat, then a longer duration would be desirable. Duration is an important factor in determining caloric expenditure. To increase caloric expenditure, it is preferable to

40

modify the duration rather than the intensity. If duration is to be extended, activities should be chosen which are orthopedically gentle.

The recommended duration of aerobic exercise is 20 to 60 minutes. Twenty minutes is a minimum requirement to improve aerobic capacity. The duration of higher-impact modes should gradually progress to a limit of 30 or 40 minutes. For low-impact activities, duration may progress to 60 minutes or even longer in some cases.

Any soreness that develops as the result of exercise should be given prompt attention. *Pain or soreness indicates that something is wrong.* Don't exercise with pain. Seek medical attention to determine the cause of the problem as well as a recommendation for treatment and future activity.

For many people, improved fitness permits involvement in new activities. For example, bicycle touring, long-distance running and cross-country ski touring are becoming increasingly popular in many age groups. These activities are not possible for the sedentary individual.

If an activity of longer duration is anticipated, it is important to increase training duration gradually in the weeks prior to the event. Training should include one or two days per week in which duration gradually becomes much longer. Before and after every relatively hard day, there should be an easy day. With proper preparation, participation in endurance events may add enjoyment to life which relatively few people have the ability or opportunity to experience.

Frequency

As with duration, the recommended weekly frequency of aerobic exercise depends in part upon the mode of activity and the goals established for the program. Some people enjoy exercise every day, while others prefer a more limited exercise program. When health benefits represent the most important reason for exercise, the activity need not be done every day.

Low-impact exercise can be performed daily, if desired, with minimal risk for overuse injuries. Higher-impact activities such as jogging or dance-exercise may require a rest day between exercise sessions. A low-impact mode of activity can be considered during the in-between days. With adequate time and appropriate progression, many individuals who wish to jog or dance-exercise daily may do so with minimal risk. As previously mentioned, immediate attention should be given to any developing soreness in order to prevent an overuse injury.

If, in addition to an improved aerobic capacity, a reduction of body fat is desired, then a more frequent exercise program may be selected. Aerobic exercise is an extremely important component of a program to reduce body fat. For fat reduction, more frequent stimulation of metabolism is helpful.

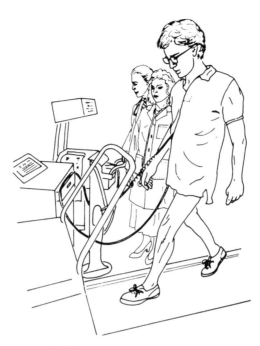

The generally recommended frequency of aerobic exercise is three to five times per week. A frequency of less than three is unlikely to result in measurable improvement. A frequency of more than five may increase the risk of overuse injuries, especially in the higher-impact modes, and provide diminishing returns related to fitness. Aerobic exercise performed at least every second day is desirable. However, for fat reduction, greater frequency is indicated. If exercise is to be performed six or seven days per week, it may be very desirable to utilize more than one mode of activity. Boredom and overuse injuries are less likely to occur with a variety of activities. Selection of more than one high-impact mode of activity is not recommended if exercise is performed six or seven days per week. Individual differences exist in the number of exercise days which may be well-tolerated. As an aerobic exercise program is established, abilities and limitations will become apparent.

Intensity

The human heart serves as a built-in exercise computer which indicates intensity. Any random group of people will exhibit many different heart rate responses to an identical workload. Heart rate (a physiological indicator of work), not speed of movement, should be the most important indicator of intensity.

Several formulas have been developed to determine the desirable heart rate for aerobic exercise. A simple and commonly used formula indicates that the desirable aerobic exercise heart rate is 70% to 85% of the maximal heart rate. There may be difficulty in determining the maximal heart rate. The most valid method is to have a maximal treadmill test in which workload is gradually increased from a low workload to a maximal workload. As a result of this test, maximal heart rate and other important information are determined.

If a treadmill test is not completed, a calculation can be made to predict maximal heart rate. This calculation predicts that maximal heart rate will be 220 minus an individual's age. Therefore, for a person who is forty years of age, the predicted maximal heart rate would be 180 beats per minute. The desirable aerobic exercise heart rate range would be 70% of 180 to 85% of 180 or 126 to 153 beats per minute. The aerobic exercise workload which produces a heart rate in this range would be appropriate. In initiating an aerobic exercise program, it is desirable to keep heart rate nearer 70%, rather than 85%, of the maximum.

Table 3.15
Exercise Heart Rate Range by Age Category

AGE	70% beat/min	85% beat/min
20	140	170
25	137	165
30	133	161
35	130	157
40	126	153
45	123	148
50	119	144
55	116	140
60	112	136
65	109	131

The use of heart rate in making judgments regarding appropriate intensity is not absolute. Medications and certain health problems may influence heart rate response. Also, because of individual differences in maximal heart rate, for some people the calculation will not be accurate. Finally, the skill of measuring heart rate requires practice and initially may be inaccurate. Therefore, additional criteria should be used in making decisions about exercise intensity.

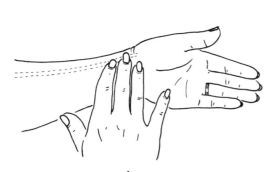

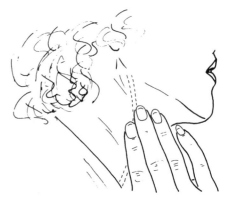

Figure 3.16 Measurement of heart rate at the radial artery.

Figure 3.17 Measurement of heart rate at the carotid artery.

The Borg Scale was developed as another method of determining exercise intensity. This scale allows quantification of an individual's perception of exercise intensity. The Borg Scale, as originally developed, is shown below:

The Borg Scale of Perceived Exertion

6
7 very, very light
8
9 very light
10
11 fairly light
12
13 somewhat hard
14
15 hard
16
17 very hard
18
19 extremely hard
20

For purposes of aerobic exercise, the intensity of exercise should not exceed 12 or 13 on the Borg Scale. Moderate, not light or not hard, are other descriptions of aerobic exercise intensity which are appropriate.

Another method to determine desirable exercise intensity is referred to as the *talk test*. If an exerciser is unable to carry on a conversation with a partner, the intensity is too high.

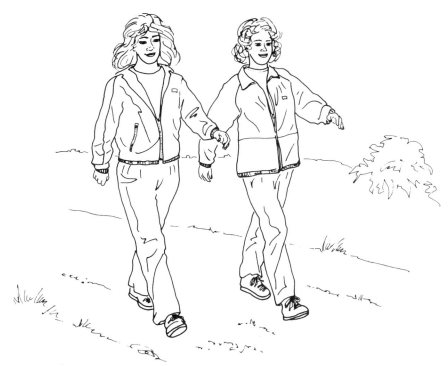

An aerobic exercise prescription can be briefly summarized as follows:

    a. Exercise at least every second day

    b. Exercise aerobically for 30 to 40 minutes per session

    c. Exercise at a moderate intensity

III. Cool Down

A cool-down period is an important component of an aerobic exercise program. Im-mediately following aerobic exercise, rhythmic movement should be maintained at a gradually reduced intensity.

During aerobic exercise, the heart pumps large quantities of blood into arteries to be delivered to working muscles. The adequate return of blood to the heart through veins requires some biomechanical assistance. Rhythmic contraction of large muscles tends to compress the soft, pliable veins which carry blood under low pressure back to the heart. Veins contain many one-way valves which permit blood to travel only in one direction. Therefore, as the veins are rhythmically compressed by large exercising muscles, blood is effectively facilitated back to the heart.

If immediately following aerobic exercise sudden cessation of activity occurs, then this skeletal muscle pump is turned off. Blood flow back to the heart is compromised as the heart continues attempts to pump large volumes of blood. If the heart receives diminishing amounts of blood, output is reduced. Ultimately, a lack of blood flow and oxygen to some parts of the body can occur. Significant cardiovascular complications can occur as the result of an insufficient cool down. For some individuals, complications could include irregular heart rhythm, loss of consciousness or a heart attack.

The consequences of an inadequate cool down can be prevented by maintaining rhythmic movement for two or three minutes following aerobic exercise. A general guideline for the cool-down period is to maintain the same activity at a gradually reduced intensity. Most importantly, following aerobic exercise, don't stop moving immediately.

It should be pointed out that stretching exercises have not been included in the recommendations for warm-up or cool down. A review of research in exercise physiology fails to provide adequate support for the need to stretch immediately prior to aerobic exercise. It is *unclear* that such stretching done prior to aerobic exercise provides protection from injury. Stretching is an important activity to improve or maintain range of motion (ROM). Good ROM may help to prevent injuries, but performing stretching exercises immediately prior to activity is not a requirement.

Evidence tends to support recommendations to stretch warm muscles rather than cold muscles. When muscle temperature increases, range of motion is enhanced. Therefore, a good time to perform stretching exercises is *immediately following* cool down. High-impact activities such as running and dance-exercise may cause a reduction in range of motion at some joints. Stretching may help to re-establish range of motion. Following aerobic exercise, muscles, especially overstressed muscles, may be in a state of mild spasm. It has been theorized that mild spasm may lead to muscle soreness experienced during the next day or two. Evidence supports the concept that gentle range-of-motion activities may help to reduce the state of mild spasm and the degree of muscle soreness which tends to follow.

Flexibility

Flexibility (range of motion) depends upon the condition and inter-relationship of bones, ligaments, muscles and tendons. Static flexibility exercises improve the range of motion of tendons and muscles by increasing elasticity and/or length. Body joints which rarely move through a complete ROM may lose flexibility. Age can also influence ROM, especially when coupled with inactivity. Conversely, appropriate flexibility exercises tend to maintain or improve ROM.

An exercise which stretches ligaments is not desirable. Loose ligaments may improve range of motion, but decrease joint stability. Therefore, squatting motions or knee flexion which cause the heel to be brought close to the buttocks would tend to stretch ligaments and destabilize the knee. People who have loose joint ligaments, caused either by inappropriate exercise or heredity, are at higher risk for joint injury and possibly other joint-related problems.

Some modes of exercise clearly enhance ROM in specific joints. For example, crawl stroke swimming can improve range of motion of the shoulder girdle. Conversely, some modes of exercise can reduce ROM. Jogging and dance-exercise can reduce ROM of the lower back, hamstrings, quadriceps and the gastroc-soleus complex (calves). Therefore, emphasis should be placed on ROM exercises for these areas.

It seems logical that performance of stretching exercises immediately prior to aerobic exercise would tend to reduce the risk of an exercise-induced injury. This concept is the premise of many warm-up regimens. However, as previously stated, evidence to support this position is lacking. At best, there is a weak relationship between *pre-exercise* stretching and injury prevention.

Ballistic Stretching and the Stretch Reflex

Ballistic stretching involves rapid or bouncy range of motion exercises. This type of stretching is generally contraindicated. Ballistic stretching does improve ROM, but can cause minute tears of muscle and tendon. Furthermore, ballistic stretching tends to evoke a stretch reflex.

Sensory receptors, known as muscle spindles, detect changes in the tension and length of muscle fibers. The main function of the muscle spindle is to respond to excessive stretching through reflex action and initiate a contraction to reduce the stretch. A rapid or extreme stretch is more likely than a static stretch to result in a stretch reflex. In a static stretch, the muscle is lengthened slowly and held for 10 to 30 seconds. Therefore, long static ROM exercises are recommended while ballistic ROM exercises should be avoided. Exercise participants should avoid painful stretching. Stretches which cause pain are clearly excessive.

Guidelines for Aerobic Exercise

In concluding this chapter, guidelines for the structure of an exercise hour are offered. The following is a description of segments which may be included in exercise classes.

Pre-Stretch Warm-Up (3–5 minutes)

The purpose of this initial segment is to warm muscles prior to stretching. This is necessary only when stretching is done prior to aerobic exercise. Suggested activities include walking, which gradually becomes brisk walking. Heart rate attained during this segment need not reach the exercise heart rate range.

Optional: Stretching and Floor Exercise (Calisthenics: 15–20 minutes)

Ballistic or bouncy stretching and so-called "toning" exercises should not be emphasized. Each movement should have an identifiable purpose, such as improvement of flexibility, muscular strength or muscular endurance.

Most movements which involve a stretch should be done slowly and held for 5–30 seconds. Most stretches should be held longer than 10 seconds. The importance of performing movements which are painless should be emphasized. The presence of pain, in any segment of the exercise session, should be discouraged. All movements should be done as safely as is reasonably possible and have a specific purpose.

Undesirable body contours are usually the result of excess fat, rather than poor muscle tone. So-called "toning," "regional" and "spot reducing" exercises do not reduce fat and, as typically done in dance-exercise, are unlikely to improve muscle tone. Aerobic exercise is the form of activity most likely to reduce body fat and improve body contour. Therefore, calisthenic movements which are of low intensity and involve many repetitions are of limited value.

Transition to Aerobic Exercise (3–4 minutes)

This segment of the exercise session represents the true warm-up. The purpose of warm-up for aerobic exercise is to gradually increase heart rate. Therefore, slow movements and low-impact activity which simulate the motions to be performed during the aerobic portion of the session are recommended.

Aerobic Exercise (20–50 minutes)

This segment should be the main focus of the exercise hour. Heart rates are usually the highest during this time. It is important to measure heart rate several times during the aerobic period, especially during the early weeks of an exercise program. These are the only times that movement should be stopped. A heart rate measurement should require a break from exercise of not more than 10 or 15 seconds. Correct measurement of exercise heart rate requires practice. Remember that the Borg Scale and the talk test are other methods of determining exercise intensity.

Cool-Down (2–3 minutes)

The purpose of cool-down from aerobic exercise is to gradually reduce heart rate while maintaining venous return of blood to the heart. It is important to maintain continuous motion during the cool-down period.

Post Cool-Down Stretch (5–10 minutes)

Stretching after aerobic exercise may be more important than stretching performed before the activity begins. The impact, weight-bearing nature of jogging and dance-exercise can reduce range of motion in the lower back, hamstrings, quadriceps and calves. These body areas should be gently stretched, following the activity, to maintain or improve range of motion. In this segment, stretches should be static and should be held for 15–30 seconds each.

Chapter Summary

- Exercise is an important part of a healthy lifestyle.
- Exercise can enhance appearance.
- Exercise can help to prevent adult atrophy.
- Exercise can help people in their sixties and beyond to be more functional.
- In the development of an exercise session or program, each exercise should be designed to measurably improve muscular strength, muscular endurance, aerobic capacity or flexibility.
- Exercises which tend to enhance muscle shape or tone are those which improve muscular strength and muscular endurance.
- "The burn" is associated with anaerobic metabolism and does not necessarily provide special benefits.
- The principles of overload and progressive resistance are important in the design of an exercise program.
- While both men and women can improve muscular strength and muscular endurance, men are likely to increase muscle size.
- Very successful competitive female body builders have body compositions which are, at least in part, genetically determined. These women are not examples of what the typical female will experience through weightlifting.
- Most aerobic activities emphasize the lower body and neglect upper body conditioning.

- If an exercise which is intended to improve muscular strength and muscular endurance can be performed with more than 25 repetitions, the resistance or load should be increased.
- The valsalva maneuver should be avoided.
- The ability to perform aerobically is a function of oxygen utilization.
- The ability of successful competitive endurance athletes is, at least in part, genetically determined.
- Aerobic capacity can be improved through aerobic exercise.
- A session of aerobic exercise should include adequate warm-up and cool-down.
- Walking is an excellent mode of aerobic exercise.
- Generally speaking, aerobic exercise should be performed every second day, at a moderate intensity, for 30 to 40 minutes.
- Range of motion is an important component of fitness.
- Ballistic stretching is generally contraindicated.

CHAPTER 4

Safe Exercise
Screening For
Those At Risk

The staff of the Meadow Brook Health Enhancement Institute strongly recommends health risk screening of all people who exercise. A review of an individual's health risk profile can help to reduce the possibility that a high-risk individual will have an exercise-related problem. In addition, risk factor screening can develop awareness of lifestyle factors which contribute to good and poor health.

According to the American College of Sports Medicine, potential exercisers can be classified according to risk profile and age. The first group is composed of individuals who are apparently healthy. These are individuals who have no symptoms and have no major coronary risk factors. People in this group are considered to be at low risk for an exercise-related problem. However, many clinicians recommend that all exercisers who are 45 years of age or older complete a maximal treadmill test regardless of risk profile.

The second group is composed of individuals at higher risk for an exercise-related problem. These are people who have symptoms suggestive of cardiovascular disease and/or at least one major coronary risk factor. For these individuals, evaluation by a physician is recommended before the initiation of an exercise program.

The third group is composed of individuals with disease. These are people with known cardiac, pulmonary or metabolic (diabetes) disease. These people should not exercise in the typical exercise setting.

Who Should Have A Maximal Exercise Test?

The American College of Sports Medicine recommends that all individuals over age 45 have a maximal exercise test before beginning an exercise program. This test is conducted by a clinician, for the purpose of identifying those who may have cardiovascular disorders which would make exercise unsafe. It is also recommended that individuals over age 35 with at least one major coronary risk factor, or anyone with symptoms of cardiovascular disease, have a maximal exercise test before beginning an exercise program. Participants of exercise programs should be made more aware of these recommendations.

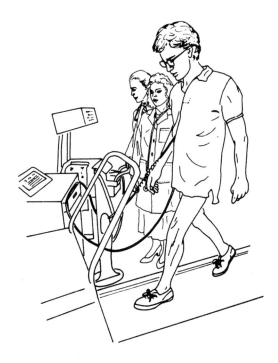

Major Coronary Risk Factors *

Research has shown that individuals who have any of the major coronary risk factors listed below are at higher risk for the occurrence of a cardiovascular event such as a heart attack or stroke. Some of these risk factors are controllable through life-style modifications.

1. History of high blood pressure (above 145/95).
2. Elevated total cholesterol/high density lipoprotein cholesterol ratio (above 5.0).
3. Cigarette smoking.
4. Abnormal resting ECG including evidence of old myocardial infarction, left ventricular hypertrophy, ischemia, conduction defects and dysrhythmias.

*Reference: Guidelines for Exercise Testing and Prescription, Third Edition, The American College of Sports Medicine, 1986, Lea & Febiger, Philadelphia, PA.

5. Family history of coronary or other atherosclerotic disease prior to age 50.
6. Diabetes mellitus.

Physical Activity Readiness Questionnaire (PAR-Q)*

For most people, physical activity should not pose any problem or hazard. PAR-Q has been designed to identify the small number of adults for whom physical activity might be inappropriate or those who should have medical advice concerning the type of activity most suitable for them.

1. Has your doctor ever said you have heart trouble?
2. Do you frequently suffer from pains in your chest?
3. Do you often feel faint or have spells of severe dizziness?
4. Has a doctor ever told you that you have a bone or joint problem, such as arthritis, that has been aggravated by exercise or might be made worse with exercise?
5. Is there a good physical reason, not mentioned here, why you should not follow an activity program, even if you wanted to?
6. Are you over age 65 and not accustomed to vigorous exercise?

If a person answers yes to any question, vigorous exercise should be postponed. Medical clearance may be necessary.

Screening Procedure

A health risk appraisal should include the following components:

1. measurement of blood pressure
2. measurement of cholesterol/HDL ratio
3. determination of history of smoking
4. determination of history of diabetes
5. analysis of body composition (percent body fat)

*Reference: PAR-Q Validation Report, British Columbia Department of Health, June, 1975, (modified version)

Blood Pressure

Measurement of resting blood pressure of all potential exercise participants is essential. Values above 140/90 are considered hypertensive. Hypertension (high blood pressure) is a primary risk factor for cardiovascular disease. Those with values above 145/95 are at higher risk and should not exercise until further evaluation has been completed by a physician.

A blood pressure of 120/80 or less is considered desirable. Low blood pressure is desirable in healthy individuals. Low blood pressure is associated with lower risk for disorders related to hypertension, like heart attack, stroke and kidney disease.

Blood pressure measurements are reported as two numbers. The first and highest, called systolic blood pressure, indicates the pressure in arteries created by contraction of the heart. The wave of pressure caused by this contraction is felt as a pulse beat at the radial artery near the wrist. The second and smaller number, called diastolic blood pressure, is the pressure which remains in arteries during the heart's resting and refilling period.

A number of lifestyle factors are related to hypertension. These include:

- excessive sodium consumption (greater than 2000 mg/day)
- excess body fat
- excessive alcohol consumption
- poorly-managed psychological stress
- inadequate aerobic exercise

Many people who don't use the salt shaker and who don't add salt in cooking may consume 6,000 to 10,000 mg of sodium per day. Ingredient lists should be read and daily totals should be quantified to determine the amount of sodium in the diet.

The skill of blood pressure measurement is relatively easy to develop. The required equipment costs about $35.00 and is available at any medical supply company. Training is often available from the community education department or nursing education department at a local hospital. Other possibilities include county health departments, the American Red Cross, or acquaintances who have been properly trained.

Cholesterol/HDL Ratio

Cholesterol is a lipid, or fat-like material, produced by all animals. All animal food products contain cholesterol. Cholesterol is produced in the human body and is essential in hormone production and cell membrane integrity. However, when too much cholesterol circulates in the blood stream, atherosclerosis, the disease process of coronary artery disease and most strokes, is accelerated. The process of atherosclerosis may begin in childhood. The rate of progression is determined by heredity and lifestyle. The lifestyle factor which most strongly influences the amount of blood cholesterol is the consumption of saturated fat. Other lifestyle factors include excess body fat and excess dietary cholesterol. However, the consumption of dietary cholesterol is not nearly as important as the consumption of saturated fat. *Foods high in saturated fat include red meats, whole dairy products, deep-fried foods and many snack foods.* Ingredient lists should be read and reviewed for fat content. Coconut oil, palm oil, palm-kernel oil, and hydrogenated oils or shortening are major sources of saturated fat, and should be avoided. Coconut oil and palm kernel oil have twice the saturated fat of beef lard. Cholesterol comes only from animals. Saturated fat comes from both plants and animals.

Cholesterol is a fatty (lipid) material which cannot dissolve directly into blood because blood is mostly water. In the body, cholesterol is combined with protein and, in this form, is water soluble. This combination of cholesterol and protein is called a lipoprotein. There are several types of lipoproteins. High density lipoprotein (HDL), the so-called good cholesterol, and low density lipoprotein (LDL), the so-called bad cholesterol, are two of the most important. HDL is considered good because it helps prevent the progression of atherosclerosis. Only a part of the total cholesterol is HDL cholesterol. Most of the remainder is LDL cholesterol, which is known promote atherosclerosis. Research has shown that the total cholesterol/HDL ratio is the most important predictor of coronary artery disease. This ratio of total cholesterol to HDL cholesterol is determined by dividing the total cholesterol number by the HDL cholesterol number. Values of 3.4 or less for males and 3.3 or less for females are considered desirable for the prevention of cardiovascular disease. Values above 5.0 place the individual at higher risk. If only a blood cholesterol value is available, values of 170 or less are considered desirable, while people with values above 200 are considered to be at higher risk. Approximately half of all Americans who die each year, have succumbed to cardiovascular diseases.

To obtain the cholesterol/HDL ratio, a blood sample must be taken. Blood samples can be drawn by making arrangements with a laboratory, health program, county health department, physician or hospital community education program in your area. Arrangements can be made for individuals or groups to have blood drawn at a nominal cost. If blood studies have been completed within one year preceding the initiation of exercise, this cholesterol/HDL ratio will be sufficient to determine risk for exercise.

If an immediate family member has a history of cardiovascular disease, a tendency toward elevated cholesterol may exist. Furthermore, if the participant consumes more than three servings per day (21 servings per week) of foods high in saturated fat (see chapter 7), then it is likely that the cholesterol/HDL ratio has been unfavorably influenced.

Smoking

If a person has not smoked for at least one month, pledges not to smoke again and has a lifetime history of less than 30 pack-years, that person can be considered at low risk for this factor. The number of pack-years is determined by multiplying the number of packs of cigarettes smoked per day by the number of years smoked. Those who smoke are considered to be at high risk.

There is no question that smoking is the single most preventable cause of death. If you can help a family member or friend to quit, you become, literally, a lifesaver.

Diabetes

Diabetes is a disorder in which blood sugar becomes elevated. This condition has a detrimental effect on every system of the body, including the cardiovascular system. A personal history of diabetes increases risk for cardiovascular disorders. Individuals with diabetes must be evaluated by a physician prior to exercise.

Diabetes tends to occur more frequently in certain families. Symptoms include excess thirst, frequent urination, fatigue, lethargy, frequent infections, slow healing as well as changes in the odor of one's breath. Lifestyle factors include excess body fat. For those with a family history of diabetes, it is very important to maintain a desirable body composition.

Health and Exercise Risk Appraisal

The following is a health and exercise risk appraisal which may be used to determine the relative safety of exercise. Its use is strongly encouraged.

Name _____ Date _____

Height _____ Weight_____ Resting Blood Pressure _____

Cholesterol/HDL Ratio _____ Number of Yes Answers _____

Primary Risk Factors of Cardiovascular Disease

Yes   *No*

1. ***Blood Pressure***
____   ____   a. Do you have a history of high blood pressure (above 145/95)?

____   ____   b. Is your resting blood pressure, as measured today, above 145/95 (either number)?

2. ***Blood Lipids*** (fats)
____   ____   a. Do you have a total cholesterol/HDL cholesterol ratio above 5.0?

Answer "b" & "c" only if "a" is not known.

____   ____   b. Do you have a family history of cardiovascular disease (heart attack, stroke, by-pass surgery, angioplasty or other evidence of disease) in siblings, parents, aunts, uncles or grandparents under age 50?

____   ____   c. Do you consume 3 servings per day (21 per week) of foods which contain large amounts of saturated fat (red meats, *whole* dairy products, deep fried foods or snack foods containing coconut oil, palm oil, palm kernel oil, hydrogenated vegetable oil or shortening)?

3. ***Smoking***
____   ____   a. Do you smoke now?

____   ____   b. Have you smoked within the last month?

____   ____   c. Do you have a smoking history of more than 30 pack-years? (Pack-years = number of packs per day times number of years smoked.)

4. *Electrocardiogram*

_____ _____   a. Do you have a history of an abnormal resting ECG including evidence of old myocardial infarction (heart attack), left ventricular hypertrophy (enlarged heart), ischemia (poor coronary circulation), conduction defects (bundle branch blocks or others), dysrhythmias (irregular heart beat)?

5. *Diabetes*

_____ _____   a. Do you have diabetes (high blood sugar)?

If a person answers yes to any of the above, then further evaluation before initiating an exercise program is recommended.

Physical Activity Readiness Questionnaire (PAR-Q)*

For most people, physical activity should not pose any problem or hazard. PAR-Q has been designed to identify the small number of adults for whom physical activity might be appropriate or those who should have medical advice concerning the type of activity most suitable for them.

Yes	*No*	
_____	_____	6. Has you doctor ever said you have heart trouble?
_____	_____	7. Do you frequently suffer from pains in your chest?
_____	_____	8. Do you often feel faint or have spells of severe dizziness?
_____	_____	9. Has a doctor ever told you that you have a bone or joint problem such as arthritis that has been aggravated by exercise, or might be made worse with exercise?
_____	_____	10. Is there a good physical reason, not mentioned here, why you should not follow an activity program even if you wanted to?
_____	_____	11. Are you over age 65 and not accustomed to vigorous exercise?

If a person answers yes to any question, exercise should be postponed. Medical clearance may be necessary.

*Reference: PAR-Q Validation Report, British Columbia Department of Health, June, 1975 (modified version).

CHAPTER 5

Recommended and Contraindicated Exercises

The following guidelines will help to create a relatively safe and effective exercise program. These guidelines apply to all classifications of individuals, including those in cardiac rehabilitation programs, diabetic health enhancement programs, wellness programs and dance-exercise groups.

1. All calisthenic exercise should have at least one of three *identifiable* purposes which follow:

    a. range of motion (flexibility)
    b. muscular endurance
    c. muscular strength

2. Ballistic stretching (rapid or bouncy) is generally contraindicated. Stretching regimens should include static stretches which are held for 10 to 30 seconds. Some range of motion exercises may be better done with slow movement such as those involving the arms and neck.
3. Stretches should be selected which are suitable for a wide variety of ranges of motion. Some anatomical positions are very difficult for certain people to assume. As a result, the position is often adapted in an undesirable manner. For example, some individuals have difficulty properly performing the modified hurdler's stretch (back of thigh stretch). The adaptation usually involves spinal flexion (forward curvature) in order to reach the lower leg. A hamstring stretch, which may be more accommodating, especially for older or obese groups, is done while lying on the back. See Figures 5.1 through 5.7.

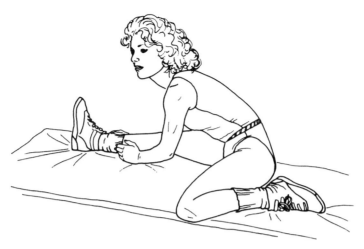

Figure 5.1 The Hurdler's Stretch. This stretch is not recommended because of the tension placed on the ligaments of the flexed knee.

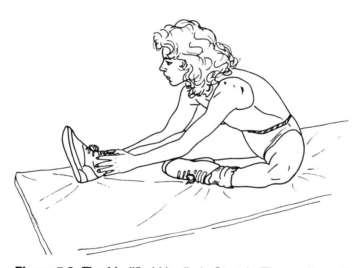

Figure 5.2 The Modified Hurdler's Stretch. The position of the flexed knee makes this stretch more desirable. However, due to lack of range of motion (flexibility) in some people, this stretch may be undesirable.

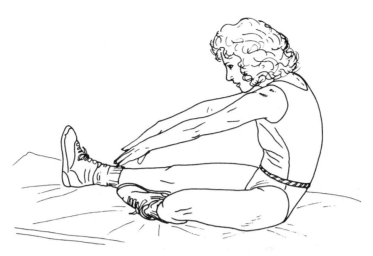

Figure 5.3 This is an undesirable adaptation of the modified hurdler's stretch. The spinal curvature demonstrates a lack of flexibility.

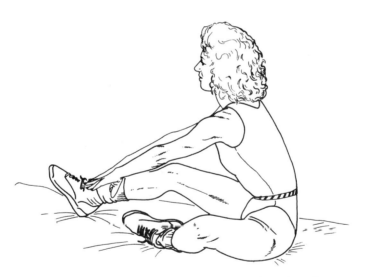

Figure 5.4 For people with limited range of motion, the modified hurdler's stretch may be performed by flexing slightly the extended leg.

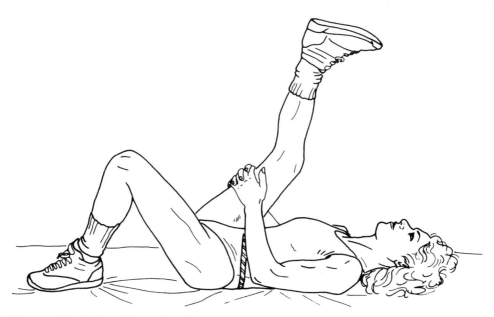

Figure 5.5 Supine Hamstring Stretch. This stretch can be performed safely by individuals with limited range of motion. With the knee held near the chest, the leg is extended to create the stretch.

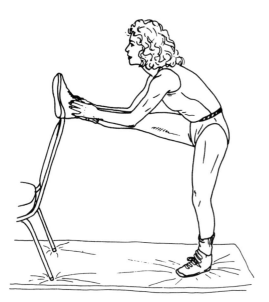

Figure 5.6a This hamstring stretch is excessive for most people. The elevated leg is too high.

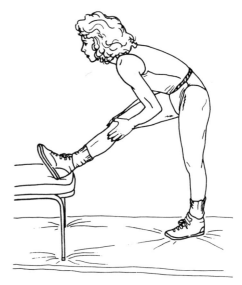

Figure 5.6b This hamstring stretch is preferred to the one shown in Fig. 5.6a. The knee of the elevated leg should be at least slightly flexed.

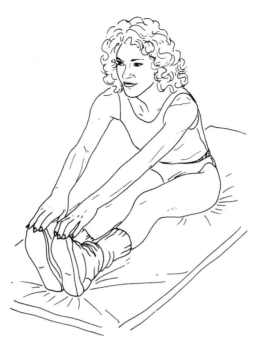

Figure 5.7 This hamstring stretch is not recommended for most people. Stretching one leg at a time is preferred. This type of foreward flexion may aggravate lower back problems.

4. Four areas which should be stretched following exercise, especially weight-bearing activity, are:

    a. lower back (Fig. 5.8)
    b. hamstrings (back of thigh) (Fig. 5.5)
    c. quadriceps (front of thigh) (Fig. 5.9)
    d. calves (back of lower leg) (Fig. 5.10)

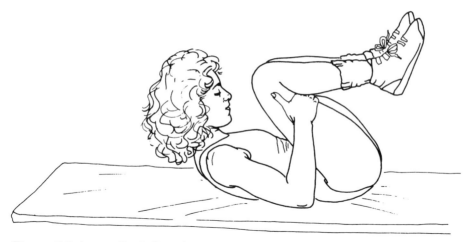

Figure 5.8 Lower Back Stretch.

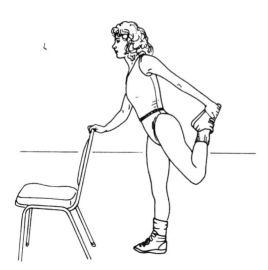

Figure 5.9 Quadriceps Stretch. The knee should not be flexed so that the heel touches the buttocks. Excess flexion could place too much tension on the ligaments of the knee.

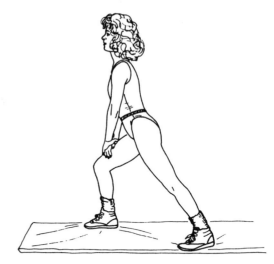

Figure 5.10 Calf Stretch. The toes of the rear foot should point directly forward.

5. Areas which can be trained for strength and endurance without equipment are:

    a. the arms and pectoral region (example: push-ups)
    b. the abdominal region (example: trunk curls)
    c. lower back (example: prone trunk lifts)

Though no equipment is required for these exercises, proper use of good equipment found in many exercise facilities is generally more effective. See Figures 5.11, 5.12, 5.13, 5.14, 5.15, 5.16 and 5.17.

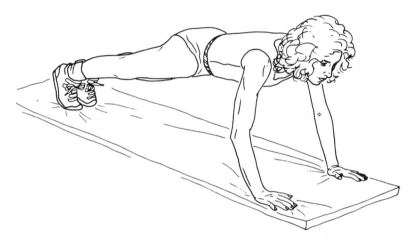

Figure 5.11 Standard Push-up. The body should be held straight.

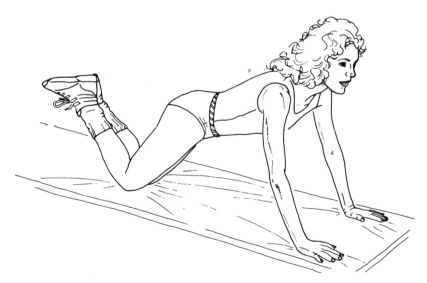

Figure 5.12 Modified Push-up. Push-ups done from the knees are for anyone who cannot yet perform standard push-ups.

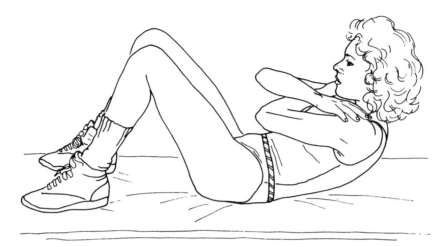

Figure 5.13 Trunk Curls. The flexing of the spine is performed by the abdominal muscles. The remainder of a complete sit-up is done by the hip flexors. The later portion of the sit-up is not necessary.

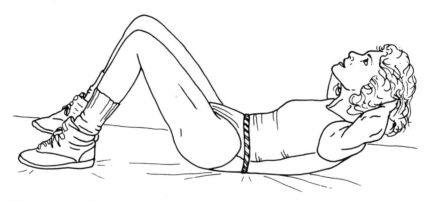

Figure 5.14 Trunk Curls. This positon is also acceptable. Note the position of the chin.

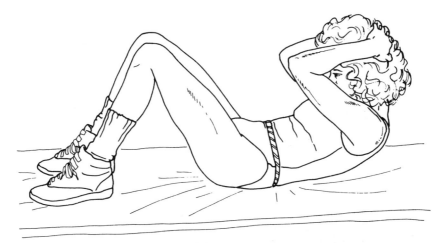

Figure 5.15 Trunk curls. This position is not recommended because of the possibility of excess flexion of the neck.

Application of biomechanical principles suggests avoidance of spinal hyperextension, especially under load. Trunk lifts done from a lying prone position may be undesirable, especially for someone with a back problem. This exercise can be made safer by maintaining contact between the feet and the floor. This reduces the possibility of hyperextension when exercising the erector spinae muscle groups. Use of back extension machines found in many exercise facilities is recommended and helps prevent low back pain. See Figures 5-16 and 5-17.

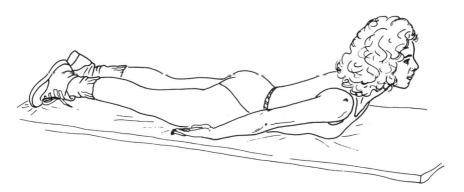

Figure 5.16 Prone Trunk Lifts. Feet should remain in contact with the floor to prevent hyperextension of the back. For additional resistance, hands may be held behind the head.

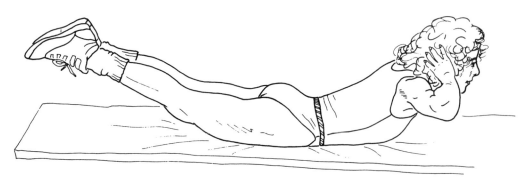

Figure 5.17 This position is not recommended. For some people, this could cause back problems.

6. It is important to be aware of inappropriate body position while exercising. (Example: Sit-ups or any abdominal exercise should not be performed with the legs held straight). See Fig. 5.18.
7. Every exercise should be performed so that the valsalva maneuver can be avoided. Individuals should exhale during exertion, inhale during recovery and avoid making grunting sounds. Breathing should not be interrupted during exercise. See Chapter 3.
8. Stretching over a locked joint (example: the knee) should be avoided. Slight flexion (bending) should be maintained, especially at the beginning of a conditioning program.
9. Stretching should be painless. If stretching hurts, the stretch is excessive.

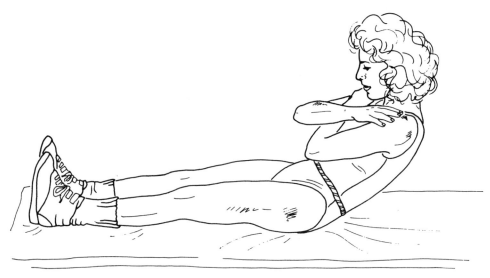

Figure 5.18 Sit-ups should not be done with straights legs.

10. Older or obese individuals should avoid leg stretches in which the legs bear weight. These positions are often difficult to hold, tend to cause an over stretch and frequently result in a valsalva maneuver. The groin stretch performed in the fencing position is an example of a stretch which these individuals should avoid. Groin muscles are more easily stretched while seated. See Figures 5.19 and 5.20.

11. The "true" hurdlers stretch is not recommended. This exercise may place excessive tension on ligaments of the flexed knee. A modification of the hurdler's stretch may be more desirable as long as the back is held straight. See Figures 5.1 through 5.7.

12. Avoidance or limitation of stretches which require standing forward flexion is desirable. These movements can place excessive tension on the ligaments of the lower back and may contribute to low-back pain. Other stretches can be selected which are more effective for the hamstrings. See Figure 5.21.

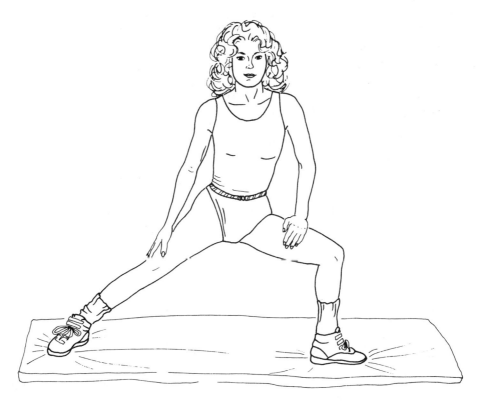

Figure 5.19 The groin stretch in the fencing position may be difficult for older or obese individuals.

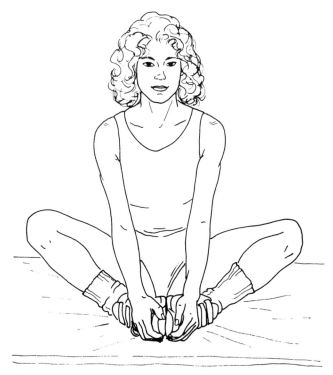

Figure 5.20 The seated groin stretch is recommended.

13. Avoid the plow. Few people can perform this stretch properly. It tends to over-stretch muscles and, for many, hyperflexes the neck under load. See Figure 5.22.

14. In exercise classes, exercise leaders should be aware of facial expressions suggestive of excessive exercise intensity. Therefore, exercise leaders should face the group at least part of the time.

15. Heart rate should be measured during the aerobic portion of exercise. Otherwise movement should be continuous during this time. If heart rates are too high, intensity should be reduced. See Chapter 3 for other recommended methods of assessing exercise intensity.

16. The aerobic portion of the exercise period should be preceded by a warm-up (transition period) designed to *gradually* increase heart rate. Warm-up can be accomplished through a gradual increase of intensity until the desired workload is reached.

17. The aerobic portion of the exercise period ideally should last 30 minutes or longer, never less than 20 minutes.

18. The aerobic portion of the exercise period should be followed by a cool-down period designed to *gradually* decrease heart rate.

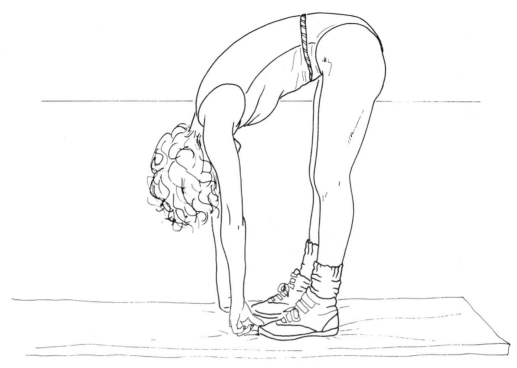

Figure 5.21 Standing forward flexion should be limited.

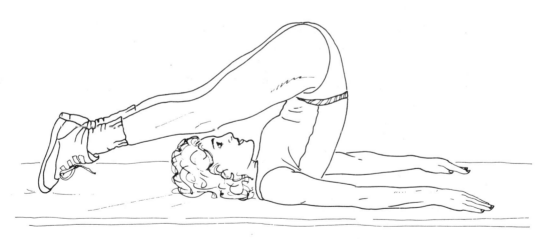

Figure 5.22 The plow is not recommended.

19. Spot reducing is not possible through regional exercise. Therefore, exercises which have been selected for this specific purpose are inappropriate.

20. Toning exercises performed on the floor represent an inappropriate use of time. Muscle tone is a state of partial contraction of a muscle at rest. Improved muscle tone does not enhance appearance when excess fat is present. Fat cannot be toned. Muscles are unlikely to demonstrate improved tone without adequate overload. Except as described in number 5 of this chapter, most floor exercises don't result in proper muscular overload. If, in the untrained state, a person can perform more than 25 repetitions of a calisthenic exercise, there is inadequate muscular overload. This type of activity is unlikely to result in improvement in muscular strength, muscular endurance or muscular toning. Even if there is proper overload, thigh exercises, for example, will not reduce and slenderize the thigh region. Most undesirable body contours are due to excess fat. Aerobic exercise is the activity which results in the greatest expenditure of calories and is most likely to result in a reduction of fat. Patterns of fat loss are hereditary.

21. Likewise, leg lifts are not recommended for toning the thigh region. Exercises to avoid include various thigh exercises such as the "hydrant" and the inner thigh leg lift. See Figures 2.1, 2.2 and 2.3.

22. Orthopedists have expressed concern about deep knee bends in which the knees are flexed more than 90 degrees. Exercises which result in hyperflexion of the knee, such that the heel touches the buttocks, also are undesirable. Consideration of both points may reduce risk of knee problems. See Figure 5.9 and 5.23.

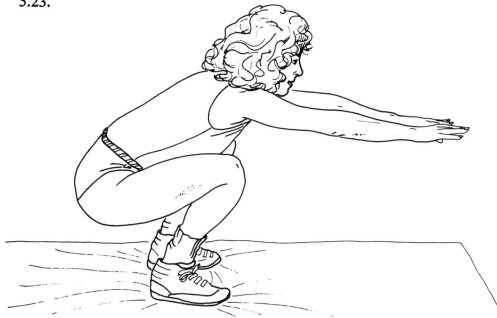

Figure 5.23 Deep knee bends are not recommended.

23. It is suggested that straight-leg abdominal exercises be avoided. These tend to cause excess lumbar extension (curvature of the lower back) which may be harmful to the spine. Exercises to avoid include various leg lifts and straight-leg sit-ups. See Figures 5.18 and 5.24.

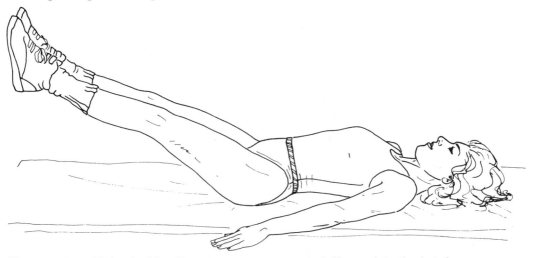

Figure 5.24a Abdominal leg lifts are not recommended. Even when the hands are held under the hips to protect the lower back (Fig. 5-24b), the abdominal muscles contract but do not shorten (isometric exercise). In this exercise, the abdominal muscles act as stabilizers as the hip flexors cause the elevation of the legs.

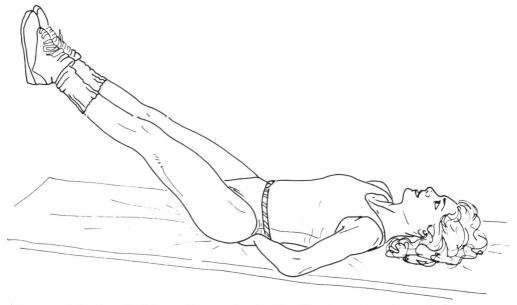

Figure 5.24b Even in this position, abdominal leg lifts are not recommended.

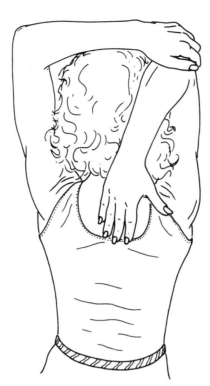

Figure 5.25 Certain stretches
for the shoulder region are
recommended. The upper body
is ignored frequently in stretching
routines.

CHAPTER 6

Fallacies of Exercise

A major objective of this book is to help the reader identify fallacies and misleading statements which appear in the media. In this chapter, common fallacies of exercise and other health-related areas are discussed. Fallacies are printed in italics.

1. *Exercise alone lowers total cholesterol in the blood and prevents heart disease.* At best, regular aerobic exercise may lower total cholesterol minimally. The reduction does not appear to be clinically significant. That is, the reduction is so minimal as not to be meaningful for the purpose of disease prevention.

    The type of cholesterol present in the blood can be altered by aerobic exercise. The HDL cholesterol (protective cholesterol) is modestly enhanced and the LDL cholesterol (harmful cholesterol) is modestly reduced. This change in the type of cholesterol present in the blood is clinically significant in the prevention of cardiovascular disease.

    It appears that the effect of exercise on the prevention of coronary heart disease is quite minimal when compared to other risk factors. Inadequate aerobic exercise is a *secondary* risk factor of coronary heart disease. Risk factors such as high cholesterol or undesirable blood lipids (blood fats), hypertension (high blood pressure), smoking and diabetes are considered to be *primary* risk factors and have a much greater influence on coronary heart disease than exercise habits. Exercise does not compensate for a fatty diet, high blood pressure or smoking. Therefore, a program of regular aerobic exercise cannot prevent coronary heart disease, regardless of the amount or type of exercise done, when primary risk factors are present.

2. *By training at high altitudes (above 8000 feet) endurance performance at sea level is enhanced.* Some running coaches continue to send their athletes to the mountains assuming that, when they come back to sea level, they will have an aerobic advantage. Scientific evidence fails to support this concept. However, if competition is to occur at a high altitude, conditioning should be conducted in a similar environment.

3. *No pain, no gain.* Exercise for health enhancement should not hurt. Painless exercise can result in excellent overall fitness. It is true that highly competitive

athletes may need to train at higher intensity for performance purposes. High intensity exercise is not a prerequisite for the achievement of health benefits nor conducive to long term participation.

4. *Feel the burn.* As described in Chapter 3, "the burn" is associated with anaerobic metabolism. The burn is not an indication that special benefits are occurring in muscle. If one stands with one arm held straight and parallel to the floor, within a minute or two the deltoid muscle of the shoulder will begin to "burn." Holding the arm in this position is unlikely to provide a fitness or toning benefit.

5. *Lactic acid causes muscle soreness the day after exercise.* Lactic acid production results from anaerobic metabolism. The pain or burning it causes lasts only as long as the activity which causes the discomfort. The mechanism associated with stiffness or soreness which may be noticed a day or two following a certain workout is not as clearly understood. Damage to the contractile filaments of the muscle, as a result of over-training, may lead to inflammation and pressure on sensory nerve endings. The sensations which follow are often described as stiffness and soreness. Light exercise seems to reduce this discomfort more effectively than no exercise.

6. *Resting heart rate is a good indicator of fitness.* In a recent issue of a fitness magazine, an article appeared which reported the physical statistics of certain fit individuals. Included were dance-exercisers, cyclists, joggers, race walkers, cross-country skiers and others. Measurements included height, weight, percent body fat, resting blood pressure and resting heart rate. The article promoted the fallacy that resting heart rate could be used to determine fitness level. It is true that some world class endurance athletes have resting heart rates in the low to mid thirties. However, many other world class endurance athletes have resting heart rates in the seventies.

   Many factors, including heredity and aerobic fitness, influence resting heart rate. When resting heart rate gradually declines over the first several weeks of regular aerobic exercise, the change is the result of improved fitness and a stronger, more efficient heart. However, the correlation between a given resting heart rate and a particular level of fitness is poor. Furthermore, an individual with a very low resting heart rate is not necessarily a good endurance athlete.

7. *Thinness is a good indicator of fitness.* Some individuals look lean and have an excellent physical appearance but don't participate in regular exercise. This observation is frustrating to those who work very hard in a training program. Appearance is a poor indicator of fitness. Even body builders who have well-defined body contours may have a poor aerobic fitness level.

8. *Stretching must precede aerobic exercise.* As described in Chapter 3, evidence that stretching immediately prior to exercise helps prevent injury or provides other benefits is inconclusive. However, activities which promote range of motion are important and seem to be most beneficial when muscles are warm.

9. *It is desirable to rock, bounce or move rhythmically during stretching movements.* As described in Chapter 3, ballistic stretching is contraindicated.

10. *It is not necessary to measure heart rate during exercise.* As described in Chapter 3, measurement of heart rate is important especially when an exercise program is initiated. Stopping or slowing movement for a few seconds to measure exercise heart rate is not likely to cause an undesirable physiological effect. While other methods of estimating exercise intensity are available, the only physiological index of exercise difficulty is heart rate.

11. *Muscle can change to fat/fat can change to muscle.* These two tissue types are very different. One tissue type can never become the other, though sometimes it may look that way. In "getting into shape" or "getting out of shape," the size of the muscle mass or fat mass may be altered. If muscle mass decreases through disuse and fat mass increases due to caloric excess, it may appear that muscle has changed to fat.

12. *"Trouble areas" may be spot reduced through exercise.* Reduction of body fat occurs when caloric expenditure exceeds caloric intake. Other than surgical removal, there is no other way. The pattern of fat loss is hereditary and cannot be altered by exercise.

13. *Body toning, body sculpting and body shaping reduce and tone flabby arms, waist and thighs.* Chapters two and three discussed this misconception extensively. This fallacy represents one of the more prevalent exercise frauds. Excess fat causes most undesirable body contours, not poorly toned muscles. Regional exercise cannot preferentially reduce body fat. Many toning routines lack sufficient overload to tone muscles. Even if effective toning is accomplished in the weight room, fat is not reshaped or reduced. Finally, there is no practical method to measure the amount of muscle tone or change in muscle tone. Therefore, perception of improvement in muscle tone is very subjective.

14. *Thigh exercises, with adequate overload, help to slenderize and tone the thighs.* Training of muscles does not make them smaller. To make the thigh smaller, fat in this region must be reduced. However, spot reduction is not possible. Thigh exercises provide only a small caloric expenditure. Aerobic exercise provides the highest caloric expenditure. Patterns of fat loss are hereditary and are not altered by exercise. Because thigh muscles are very active in lower body aerobic exercise, additional benefits obtained by performing regional thigh exercises will require much overload and time.

15. *Exercises for the waistline are helpful in eliminating love handles and the spare tire.* This is another version of the spot reducing misconception. Sit-ups are unlikely to slenderize the waistline. Abdomens protrude because of excess fat, not because of sagging muscles. It is not the rectus abdominis that hangs over the belt.

16. *Gluteal exercises firm sagging fannies.* The gluteus maximus is not likely to "droop." However, excess fat may have this appearance. This observation can be supported by identifying a subject with a "sagging fanny" and requesting a voluntary contraction of all the muscles of the gluteal region. Contracted muscle will be firm and taut, even more so than the firmness of good resting tone. Observe the region. In all likelihood, it will still sag and will continue to sag until the fat is reduced.

17. *Weightlifting is a great fat burner and body shaper.* Thirty minutes of weightlifting does not generate the caloric expenditure of thirty minutes of aerobic exercise. However, if excess fat is not present, then weightlifting may result in a reshaping of the body.

18. *Women who lift heavy weights are likely to develop large muscles.* As discussed in Chapter 3, three sessions of one hour per week, for the vast majority of females, are unlikely to create large muscles. Strength, on the other hand, may improve significantly.

19. *Ankle and hand weights are useful for developing muscular strength, muscular endurance and muscle tone.* For most people, one to three pound weights on the ankle or hands do not provide adequate muscular overload. Ankle weights used in walking or jogging may alter the mechanics of movement, may increase the impact force placed upon the lower limb and, therefore, may increase the likelihood of injury. Hand weights may be useful in walking or low impact aerobics to further elevate heart rate and increase aerobic work, if the weights are swung vigorously. Hand weights can become dangerous projectiles in group settings.

20. *Moving a light weight many times provides the same result as exercise with heavy weights.* Muscular overload is a function of muscle tension. If so little muscular tension is created than more than 25 repetitions may be performed, then the muscular overload is inadequate. The use of light weights does not result in adequate muscle tension. Regional exercise involving many repetitions is not likely to be very productive.

21. *A program of circuit weight training provides aerobic exercise.* It is incorrectly assumed that if exercise results in a sustained heart rate of 70% to 85% of maximal heart rate, that the exercise is aerobic. In fact, *anaerobic* exercise in-

terrupted by frequent short rest intervals can provide such a sustained heart rate. For exercise to be aerobic, activity must be *completely continuous.*

In circuit weight training, a series of weight machines is employed. Each machine is used for 30 seconds followed by 15 seconds of rest. During the rest period, the individuals moves to the next machine and prepares for the next 30 second exercise period. Though the exercise session may last 30 minutes, the activity is a series of anaerobic exercises, not aerobic exercise. While there are some minimal aerobic benefits, a circuit weight training program results primarily in the development of muscular endurance.

22. *Women should always do push-ups on the knees rather than the toes.* Anyone, male or female, who cannot perform push-ups on the toes should perform them on the knees. When 15 push-ups from the knees can be completed, the resistance should be increased by performing them from the toes (Principle of Progressive Resistance).

23. *Products which increase sweating during exercise, such as plastic suits or rubber garments, are beneficial in controlling weight and enhancing appearance.* Any product which enhances sweating tends to dehydrate the body, thus resulting in weight loss. The loss of body fluid (or muscle mass) during weight loss is very undesirable. Sweating, in itself, does not encourage fat loss. Exercise in minimal clothing is as effective in burning fat as exercise in heavy clothing. Furthermore, when as little as one or two pounds are lost as a result of dehydration, performance can decline and the likelihood of a heat stress disorder, such as heat stroke, increases. Heat stroke can cause brain damage, damage to other internal organs and can even cause death. For every pound of weight loss as the result of exercise, one pound (one pint) of additional fluid, in the form of water, diluted fruit juice or diluted sports drink, should be consumed. The choice of fluids depends on personal preference.

Finally, the wearing of rubberized belts or shorts does not result in the elimination of fat from "trouble spots." Spot reducing is not likely under any circumstances.

24. *Athletes and others who exercise need special foods or supplements.* Except for the need to consume 70% of all calories in the form of carbohydrates, there is little evidence to suggest that those who exercise have special nutritional needs. Consumption of special foods or supplements (including protein supplements, vitamin supplements, mineral supplements, free amino acid supplements, bee pollen supplements, lecithin supplements, ginseng supplements, evening primrose supplements, wheat germ oil supplements or any other supplement for which claims are commonly made) provide no performance benefits. Body builders have been particularly susceptible to this misconception.

25. *A diet which is especially high in protein is beneficial to bodybuilders or others who exercise.* The average American male and female consumes 200% and 150%, respectively, of the recommended dietary allowance (RDA) for protein. An objective review of research, involving the maximal amount of muscle mass which can be added to the body in one day, makes it difficult to support the consumption of more protein than is consumed by the average American. The body cannot store extra protein. Excess dietary protein adversely affects the liver, the kidneys and the bones. A high protein diet can cause the loss of extra calcium through the urine. It is very difficult to find any benefits of a high protein diet.

    The consumption of liquid or free amino acid supplements is very prevalent in body building. However, scientific evidence does not support that these materials are influential in the development of muscular hypertrophy (size). Liquid or free amino acids save the intestinal tract the task of digesting protein into its amino acid components. This is a task which the digestive tract does very well. It's like putting a healthy, functional person on crutches. However, with the amino acid supplements, the composition of the product frequently emphasizes certain amino acids in a manner which may not typically be seen in food. Those with substantial backgrounds in nutrition research and education have expressed that high doses of certain amino acids may be causing imbalances and effective shortages of other amino acids found in normal food and could possibly be detrimental over time. The long term effects are not yet clear.

    It is very difficult to convince bodybuilders that such supplements are unnecessary. Bodybuilders seem to believe the myths perpetuated by other bodybuilders. The sale of protein, amino acid and other supplements is a huge business driven by a very large profit margin. Here is another case in which tradition has been developed through the repetition of unsupported statements. As a final point, common practices involving drugs (including anabolic steroids), dehydration and supplementation make competitive body building one of the most self-abusive of all sports. Unfortunately, few competitive body builders heed the risks and possible health consequences. For those familiar with the risks, the desire to win is often more important than health.

26. *Water should not be consumed immediately before, during or immediately following exercise.* To maintain hydration and performance and to prevent heat stress disorders, water should be consumed before, during and after exercise.

27. *Vitamin supplements provide extra energy.* While vitamins act as catalysts in certain metabolic pathways which result in the production of energy, vitamins don't contain calories and therefore cannot provide energy. The best advice for athletes is to consume the recommended daily allowance (RDA) of vitamins and minerals. These guidelines include a rather large safety factor so as to be

80

adequate for nearly every reasonably healthy person. There are certainly individual differences of requirement but it is difficult to find support for consumption of vitamins or minerals in excess of the RDA. The best way to obtain vitamins is to consume them as part of a varied diet which is high in carbohydrate. This diet should include a wide variety of fruits, vegetables, whole grains, skim dairy products and legumes. The fat content should be very limited.

28. *Vitamin supplements help to prevent colds, flu and other infections.* This is certainly a controversial area of nutrition. On the one hand, a Nobel laureate and a few others claim that Vitamin C, when consumed in tens of times the RDA, provides additional immunity to colds, flu and cancer. On the other hand, countless researchers in the field of nutrition are unable to come to the same conclusion. If megadoses of Vitamin C have the effects claimed by Pauling and his supporters, then these remarkable characteristics should be easily demonstrated in a controlled research setting by nearly all those who perform research in Vitamin C. Such is not the case.

29. *Sports drinks are helpful to those who perform regular aerobic exercise.* For continuous aerobic exercise lasting less than two hours in duration, there is no particular benefit associated with the consumption of currently available sports drinks. Water is the preferred fluid for this type of exercise. Only in very long distance events, such as a marathon (run of 26.2 miles), are sports drinks likely to be beneficial.

30. *People slow down and become less functional largely due to the aging process.* Lack of appropriate activity and other lifestyle factors, rather than the biological aging process, seem to be responsible for much of the atrophy and degenerative processes seen in older individuals in the United States. There are many examples of people beyond the age of 60 who have remained adequately active. These individuals are in many ways more functional than younger sedentary people.

31. *The resting metabolic rate and the need for calories are reduced as part of the aging process.* The loss of muscle mass which results from inadequate physical activity results in a decline of resting metabolism and resting caloric expenditure. The muscle mass is more metabolically active, even at rest, than fat tissue. As the lean mass declines, caloric need may decline and the caloric excess eventually results in an increase in body fat.

32. *Chances of developing heart disease or cancer are influenced more by heredity than by lifestyle factors.* Research has shown that many chronic degenerative diseases can be prevented by appropriately altering lifestyle habits. The ability to prevent disease is clearly in our own hands. If all Americans would adequately limit dietary fat, control blood pressure, avoid

tobacco, control weight, and be adequately active, the incidence of heart disease would fall even more rapidly than it has over the past twenty years. Research has shown that the steady decline of heart disease has resulted primarily from lifestyle changes which many Americans have made.

33. *Fitness magazines provide accurate, well-researched articles and advertisements for safe, effective products.* Fitness magazines provide accurate, controversial *and* misleading information. For many people, the differentiation of accurate from misleading information is very difficult.

34. *Devices which are claimed to trim the abdomen, as advertised in magazines, tend to be effective.* These devices, which have been sold under a variety of names, consist of long springs, too foot stirrups and two hand grips. The individual in the ads is pictured sitting with hands and feet in place using the device. With the arms and legs held almost straight, the subject extends the body, stretching the springs which are held between hands and feet. The ads suggest that this exercise will firm and flatten the protruding abdomen and that this problem is the result of poorly-toned muscles. This promotes two fallacies: that protruding abdomens are caused by sagging muscles and that the extension of the springs requires the contraction of the abdominal muscles. The extension of the springs actually requires the contraction of certain back muscles, not abdominal muscles.

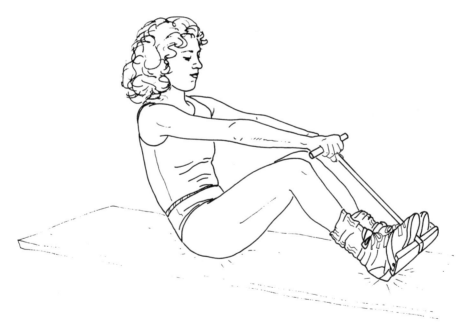

Figure 6.1 Millions of dollars are wasted annually on exercise devices like this one. Let the buyer beware of false claims.

35. *A toned muscle is smaller than a flabby muscle. A toned muscle therefore takes up less space and causes the circumference of the particular body region to be smaller.* While this misconception sounds logical, there is no evidence to support the concept. One way to test the hypothesis is to temporarily cause a muscle group to be firmer (by voluntary contraction) and measure the circumference of the region. Using the thigh or arm as an example, gently contract the muscles of the region. This gentle contraction stimulates improved resting tone and firmness. Measurements done before and after are likely to be similar.

Exercise (such as strength training) which may result in improved muscle tone doesn't make muscles smaller. If anything, such exercise make muscles slightly larger.

Undesirable flabbiness is more likely to result from excess body fat than from poorly-toned muscles. The reduction of excess body fat is the most appropriate way to decrease regional circumference.

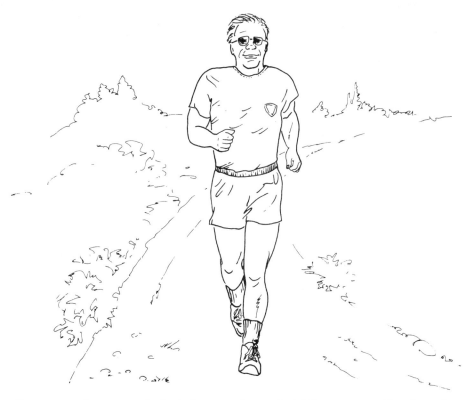

Figure 6.2 Some people in their seventies and eighties are capable of running marathons. (26 mi. plus 385 yds).

36. *For older people who demonstrate poor fitness, it is too late for exercise to result in any real benefit.* Research has demonstrated that significant physiological and psychological improvements result from a well-designed program of regular exercise, regardless of advanced age.

CHAPTER 7

Quality of Life and Body Composition
The Nutrition Connection

In addition to exercise, the pursuit of good health and physical attractiveness involves nutrition. While nutrition may play a greater role in disease prevention, both exercise and nutrition can influence body composition. Therefore, certain matters of nutrition become relevant issues.

One such issue involves the energy balance equation. It ultimately determines whether body fat increases, decreases or remains unchanged.

Table 7.1
The Energy Balance Equation

Calories Spent at Rest + Calories Spent
in Activity = Calories Consumed

As long as this statement is true for an individual, the amount of body fat will remain constant. If the statement is false for an individual, the amount of body fat will change.

A strategy to balance the equation or to help cause an imbalance in favor of the reduction of body fat is to modestly limit caloric intake. Modest limitation rather than severe limitation seems to provide the best opportunity for long term success, especially when coupled with a permanent program of regular aerobic exercise. For many Americans, a reduction of caloric intake can be accomplished without limiting the amount of food consumed. Rather, the kind of food consumed can be altered. An examination of the caloric relationship of nutrients is important to understand this concept.

Since dietary fat contains more than twice the calories of other nutrients, and alcohol, a non-nutrient, contains nearly as many calories as fat, it should be obvious which dietary components are best to avoid. Identifying sources of alcohol should not be difficult. Identifying sources of fat, however, may require more effort.

Table 7.2
The Caloric Relationship of Nutrients and Alcohol

Carbohydrate (starch or sugar)	4 calories/gram
Protein (plant or animal)	4 calories/gram
Fat (plant or animal)	9 calories/gram
Vitamins	0 calories/gram
Minerals	0 calories/gram
Water	0 calories/gram
Fiber	0 calories/gram
Alcohol	7 calories/gram

The average American consumes a large amount of fat which totals 37% to 42% of all calories consumed. By directing eating habits away from fat and toward carbohydrate, an individual could eat the same amount of food while consuming substantially fewer calories. *As well as helping to prevent obesity, the reduction of dietary fat tends to reduce the likelihood of developing coronary artery disease, stroke and cancer.* (Foods which contain much added sugar should also be avoided becuse added sugar is frequently very concentrated in foods, adding many calories with no other nutrients.) The consumption of the following foods should be reduced or eliminated.

Table 7.3
Foods Generally High in Fat

Red Meat (red before cooking)

Processed Meats (hot dogs, sausage, bacon, lunch meat)

Whole Dairy Products (whole milk, cheese, butter, ice cream, 2% milk, etc.)

Deep Fried Foods (french fries, fish, chicken, donuts, etc.)

Many Snack Foods (cookies, crackers, donuts, chips, candy, chocolate, pies, cupcakes, etc.)

Foods Which Contain: Shortening
Hydrogenated Oils
Coconut Oil
Palm Kernel Oil
Palm Oil
Other Vegetable Oils
Mayonnaise
Salad Dressing

From this list it may be assumed that all dairy products are undesirable. Skim milk, 1/2% milk, low-fat yogurts and low fat cottage cheese are highly recommended. The consumption of the following foods should be emphasized.

Table 7.4

Foods Generally High in Complex Carbohydrates (starch)
but Low in Fat and Sugar[1]

Pasta (limiting added fats, cheese or sour cream)

Rice (limiting added fats, cheese or sour cream)

Whole Grain Bread

Some Breakfast Cereals (depending on ingredients)[2]

Oatmeal

Oat Bran Cereal

Beans (Pinto, Navy, White, Great Northern, etc.)

Bread (White is less desirable than *whole* grain)

Muffins (depending on ingredients)

Dessert Breads (depending on ingredients)

Starchy Vegetables (baked potato, squash, etc.)

[1]Ingredient lists should contain little or none of the items shown on the high-fat list.
[2]Breakfast cereals should contain no more than 1 gram of fat or 3 grams of simple sugars (sucrose and other sweetners) per one-ounce serving. This information is listed on all cereal boxes under the heading "Carbohydrate Information."

Another important strategy to improve nutritional habits is to examine food labels for key information. The amount of fat which a food contains is frequently the most important imformation. However, some food producers try to hide certain nutritional facts.

For example, there are three ways to quantify the amount of fat in food. Two of these quantifications make high fat foods appear to be low in fat. The meat industry reports fat by *percent of weight.* Fast food outlets may indicate that the meat in hamburgers is only 20% fat. This value sounds low, however, the *percent of calories* from fat is approximately 66%. This value sounds high. Actually, hamburger is a major source of fat, especially saturated fat, in the American diet.

The dairy industry reports fat by *percent of volume.* Whole milk is reported to be 3 1/2% fat. This value also sounds low. However, 48% of the calories in whole milk come from fat. Whole milk is a major source of fat in the American diet, especially saturated fat.

The method which best discriminates between high-fat and low-fat foods is analysis by percent of calories. As a general rule, foods with 50% or more of their calories from fat should be consumed very infrequently. Foods which contain 20% or less of their calories from fat need not be limited because of fat content.

An example of misleading labeling is packaged lunch meat. Bold type may indicate that the product is 80% fat free by weight. The same package may also indicate that there are 70 calories per serving (1 slice) and that each serving contains 6 grams of fat. Six grams of fat contain 54 calories (6 grams times 9 calories per gram). Therefore, 54 calories of every 70 calories, or 77%, come from fat. Though labeled 80% fat free, this product is nearly 80% fat. Such products identified as 95% fat free may contain 50% of their calories in the form of fat.

Comparing Starchy and Fatty Foods

A typical fast food burger may contain 640 calories and be 56% fat. A plate of pasta with a well-seasoned, meatless tomato sauce may also contain 640 calories but could be less than 15% fat. The 640 calories of pasta would provide much more food to eat than the 640-calorie burger. Because pasta and other starches are relatively low in calories, a much larger quantity must be consumed to equal the number of calories in a burger. However, all pasta dishes are not low in calories. Many pasta salads contain so much vegetable oil that they too become high-fat foods. Fat is often so well-hidden that fatty foods may not seem fatty at all. Such is frequently the case with past salad purchased in a deli or a restaurant.

The possibility exists that excess fat calories may be more easily stored in the body than excess carbohydrate calories. Since the body's ability to store carbohydrate is limited, excess carbohydrate is converted to fat for storage. An additional energy expenditure is required to convert and store carbohydrate as fat. As much as 23% of the energy in carbohydrate may be used in this conversion process, leaving only 77% of excess carbohydrate calories which become stored as fat. Excess dietary fat, on the other hand, is easily stored, requiring only a 3% energy expenditure for this process. Therefore, 97% of excess fat (but only 77% of excess carbohydrate) appears to be stored in the body as fat.

Disease Prevention

Of all the lifestyle factors which influence the risk of developing chronic degenerative diseases, nutrition is one of the most important. The large amount of dietary fat consumed by the typical American increases the likelihood of developing atherosclerosis (a disease of arteries which leads to a heart attack or stroke) and cancer. The link between dietary fat and cancer is a relatively recent discovery.

While all dietary fats are very high in calories, only saturated fat appears to promote artery disease. The consumption of saturated fat tends to cause more cholesterol to circulate in the bloodstream. Elevated blood cholesterol can cause the process of atherosclerosis to progress more rapidly. As atherosclerosis develops, arteries, especially coronary arteries, become progressively narrower over a period of roughly 20 to 50 years. Eventually, the flow of blood through the narrowed areas is so poor that certain tissues are deprived of oxygen. In the heart or brain, when the delivery of oxygen is interrupted, a heart attack of stroke occurs. Unfortunately, there are no symptoms associated with this disease until it becomes very advanced.

Atherosclerosis may begin early in life. Because of the amount of fat consumed by American children, as well as adults, the disease is thought to begin in nearly all Americans by the age of 12. The disease initially produces fatty streaks in the arteries. This streaking does not tend to be evident in populations that have a low fat intake. Research involving American youth repeatedly indicates that large numbers of children between the ages of six and twelve have multiple risk factors of artery disease. These risk factors include elevated blood cholesterol, elevated blood pressure and obesity. Though the incidence of artery disease, especially the incidence of heart attack, has steadily decreased over the past twenty years, this trend may become less evident as high risk children progress through adulthood. Research suggests that the decline of heart disease seen in the United States has resulted from the improved lifestyle habits of adult Americans. There is general agreement that the best way to have good lifestyle habits as adults is to develop good habits in childhood. After the age of two years, it is recommended that dietary fat be restricted to no more than 30% of total caloric intake. The Meadow Brook Health Enhancement Institute has established as a goal for its adult participants, an intake of dietary fat which does not exceed 18% of total calories consumed.

Table 7.5
Dietary Recommendations of the Meadow Brook Health Enhancement Institute

Nutrient	% of Total Calories
Total Dietary Carbohydrate Emphasizing Starch, Limiting Simple Sugars	70%
Protein Emphasizing a Variety of Plant Sources	12%
Fat Utilizing Monounsaturated Fats and Polyunsaturated Fats, Limiting Saturated Fats	18%

Table 7.6
Recommended Daily Nutrition

Food Groups to Include	Servings Per Day[3]
Fruits	2
Leafy Vegetables	1
Non-leafy Vegetables	2
Whole Grain Products	2
Skim or Low-Fat Dairy Products	4
Lean Meats or, preferably, Vegetable protein sources such as legumes (dry beans, peas, lentils, some nuts, etc.)	2
	—
	13

[3]The size and number of servings per day may be influenced by one's caloric requirement.

Regardless of family history, risk factor analysis makes cardiovascular disease very *predictable*. Through adequate risk factor modification cardiovascular disease is *preventable*. See Chapter 4 for a review of risk factors.

Since thirteen servings of food per day are recommended daily and it is unlikely that all can be eaten in one meal, a total of three or more meals should be consumed per day. The thirteen servings shown in Table 7.6 represent good nutrition. Individuals who follow this plan every day are not likely to need a vitamin or mineral supplement.

The one-meal-a-day plan has not been demonstrated to be an effective method of long-term weight control. Eating one meal per day results in fasting for 23 1/2 hours per day. Such a nutritional plan may depress metabolism in response to the long hours of fasting. The ultimate result may be a reduction in the caloric requirement to maintain weight. Therefore, to prevent an increase in body fat, a reduction of caloric intake may be required.

The Set Point Theory of Weight Control

As the energy balance equation is kept in mind, the combination of modest caloric restriction through limitation of dietary fat and moderate aerobic exercise may result in an imbalance of the equation. This tends to result in a reduction of body fat. However, there is one more variable which may not remain constant. This variable is the resting metabolism. The calories required for resting metabolism are far greater than the caloric expenditure of aerobic exercise, even when exercise is performed every day for an hour. For example, an individual may require 2300 calories per day to maintain weight and may perform a brisk walk of 60 minutes every day. This person may require 1800 calories to maintain resting metabolism and 500 calories to perform activity. With this relationship in mind, something that would depress the resting metabolism by 20% or more (360 calories or more) would create a significant weight control problem. This issue is addressed by the Set Point Theory.

The Set Point Theory suggests that a mechanism in the brain regulates the amount of fat stored in the body. This mechanism works much like a thermostat which, in this case, is set at a particular amount of stored body fat. If caloric intake is restricted causing a remarkable reduction of body fat, the setting of the thermostat will tend to cause the body to conserve fuel by slowing the resting metabolic rate and therefore reducing the caloric requirement. The theory suggests that the body will continue to conserve fuel until the set point of body fat is achieved. Conversely, if too much fat is stored in the body, calorie wasting mechanisms may take effect, causing a wasting of fuel until such time as the set point is reached again. It appears that the calorie conserving mechanisms are more effective than the calorie wasting mechanisms in most Americans. However, there are individuals who are capable of eating ''practically anything'' without gaining weight. Is there a method, according to the theory, to change the setting of the thermostat? The answer seems to be yes.

Factors which tend to raise the set point, causing a gradual rise in the amount of body fat to be stored, include some typically American behaviors. These include the high-fat diet, rapid weight-loss dieting and insufficient activity. Thus, as supported by the theory, Americans tend to gain weight gradually throughout adulthood.

Factors which tend to lower the set point, causing a reduction in the amount of body fat to be stored, include the high-carbohydrate, low-fat nutritional plan, regular adequate meals and consistent aerobic exercise. Changes in the set point seem to occur over a long period of time. Therefore, long term habits affect the set point.

Recent research suggests that heredity plays an important role in determining the amount of fat to be stored in the body. Each individual apparently inherits a particular degree of difficulty related to maintaining or achieving recommended weight (percent body fat). Even though some people may inherit a genetic tendency toward obesity, such individuals should not reject good habits of nutrition and exercise. Regardless of genetic tendency, the degree of obesity can be reduced through good lifestyle habits. A few people may not reasonably be able to achieve desirable body composition, but they will be leaner as the result of permanent improvements in exercise habits, behaviors related to eating and fat content of the nutritional plan.

Fallacies of Weight Control

1. *The goal of a weight-loss program is to lose weight.*

    This may be the greatest fallacy of weight control. Primary emphasis should be placed on the reduction of *body fat* with little or no loss of the lean mass (muscle) or body fluids. Diets which tend to cause losses of lean tissue and body fluids are the ones which tend to result in the most rapid loss of *weight.* The loss of body fat generally does not occur rapidly. When the rate of weight loss exceeds one pound per week, the likelihood increases that lean tissue and body fluids account for some of the loss. Don't rely on the bathroom scale to determine the progress. The scale can not determine the amount of fat that has been lost.

2. *It is possible to permanently lose 3 to 7 pounds of fat per week in a well-designed, quick weight-loss program.*

    This is the essence of the advertised claims and testimonials but the statement is not supported by the facts. A few calculations related to a loss of five pounds of fat in one week will illustrate this point. Five pounds of fat contain 17,500 calories. To lose five pounds of fat, a deficit of 17,500 calories must be created *and* all of the deficit must come only from fat, not lean tissue. A daily deficit of 2,500 calories per day would be required. Many people don't consume 2,500 calories per day. Therefore, for many individuals a deficit of 2,500 calories per day is not possible. For others, a deficit of 2,500 calories per day would be so severe as to cause a starvation defense response resulting in a remarkable reduction of the resting metabolic rate. As the resting metabolic rate diminishes, there is a corresponding reduction of the caloric deficit and the rate of fat loss.

    One participant of a quick weight-loss program stated that she had learned to tolerate her 500 calorie diet quite well. While she was hungry at meal time, meals totaling 500 calories per day left her without severe hunger. Though she had been losing an average of one or two pounds per week without exercise, she saw her adjustment to the diet as a good sign. Feeling able to stay on the diet, she thought, was a sign of future success. With a better understanding of metabolism, she should have been quite concerned. Someone who is reasonably satisfied with 500 calories per day may have a metabolic rate that is well below average. Such a depression of metabolic rate is a common response to a very low-calorie diet. This reduction of caloric need is thought to be an important factor which influences the regaining of weight following such a diet even when reasonable eating habits are maintained.

3. *During weight loss, carbohydrate is the nutrient which should be severely limited.*

When dietary carbohydrate is severely limited, loss of body fluids occurs. Roughly one pound (454 grams) of carbohydrate, in the form of glycogen, is stored in the human body. Nearly three grams of water are stored with every gram of carbohydrate. This water is not the water which causes periodic bloating or puffiness. It is essential that this water be present for storage of carbohydrate in the body. When the body is depleted of carbohydrate through a low-carbohydrate diet, the one pound of carbohydrate and three pounds of water are quickly lost. None of this weight loss is fat.

Carbohydrate is a very important nutrient. In addition to being the preferred fuel for muscular activity, carbohydrate is the only fuel usable by the brain and other nerve cells under normal circumstances. The brain cannot use fat for fuel though many other body cells can. Since the brain has such a strong need for carbohydrate and since the storage capacity is small, a safety mechanism exists which permits production of new carbohydrate. The body cannot make new carbohydrate from fat, but new carbohydrate can be made from protein. Thus, when carbohydrate stores are low and when dietary sources are restricted, protein is scavenged from many different tissue types (mostly muscle) to make new carbohydrate. As muscle mass is diminished, the resting metabolic rate and the need for calories declines. The nutrient which can help to prevent the loss of lean mass and the reduction of resting metabolism is dietary carbohydrate. Any weight loss plan should include at least 100 grams, though preferably 150 grams, of carbohydrate. This would represent 400 to 600 carbohydrate calories per day.

4. *Advertisements for weight-loss products or programs are reasonably accurate and these advertised products or programs are safe and effective.*

Many weight loss products which have been advertised on television and in the print media have contained grossly inaccurate and misleading statements. A quick and easy method to permanently lose body fat does not exist. Therefore, claims for pills that block the digestion or absorption of food, or claims that fat will be quickly flushed or melted away, represent consumer fraud. Money-back guarantees frequently confuse consumers into believing that a product must be credible. Few people take the time to request refunds even when the product is not effective. Sometimes requests are ignored. If a product is ever developed which is helpful in promoting quick, easy and permanent weight-loss, be assured that this product will be so newsworthy as to be reported widely in the national news for weeks.

5. *Exercise is not a good method of weight-loss.*

Upon initial reflection, exercise may appear to be an inefficient method for losing weight. One pound of body fat contains 3500 calories. When a person who weighs 150 pounds jogs a mile, approximately one hundred calories are expended. Does this mean that a person has to jog 35 miles to lose one pound? Absolutely not! It is true that when a person has jogged 35 miles, the number of calories expended during the jogging is roughly the same as the number of calories found in one pound of body fat. Aerobic exercise provides weight-loss benefits in addition to the expenditure of calories during the exercise itself. (See Chart 3.1.) Dieting alone tends to depress resting metabolism.

Regular aerobic exercise is a very important component of an effective weight-control program. A program that does not include regular aerobic exercise is less likely to be successful, especially in the long term. It is important to note that excess body fat is an indication of a need for a *permanent* change in lifestyle habits. Temporary changes in behavior tend to result in only a temporary change in body fat. For approximately 85% of all people who lose weight by diet only, all the weight plus a little more is regained within a year or two. Growing evidence suggests that weight-loss dieting, especially rapid weight-loss dieting, results in a starvation defense response. As the body adapts to restricted caloric intake, metabolism becomes more efficient and the need for calories is reduced. Beware of rapid weight-loss diets! Contrary to advertised claims and testimonials, it is very unlikely that someone can lose 3 to 7 pounds *of fat* in a week. It is possible to lose 3 to 7 pounds, but body fluid and muscle mass may account for more than half the loss. To help insure that only fat is lost, the rate of weight-loss should not exceed one pound per week. At this rate, weight-loss is more likely to be permanent.

While childhood obesity is being reported more frequently, most overweight adults began their weight gain in their late teens and early twenties. The typical rate of weight gain for American adults is one to three pounds per year. Regular aerobic exercise can prevent this change of body composition. As with heart disease and cancer, the best intervention is prevention.

6. *Cellulite is a particular type of fat which is reduced through a specially designed diet, specially designed exercise and other procedures such as herbal wraps.*

   Cellulite is not a medical or scientific term. What is called cellulite is seen more often in women than men and is thought to be the result of hormonal influences, excess body fat and the nature of connective structures within fat. Chemically, it is the same as other body fat which does not look lumpy or bumpy. The specific reason for the "cottage-cheese" appearance does not seem to be clear. However, lumpy fat is reduced best by exactly the same method as is excess fat found anywhere in the body.

7. *I don't need to lose weight, I just need to redistribute my weight.*

   This kind of error may be made by using height and weight charts to determine correct weight. The percent of body fat should be the factor used to determine desirable weight. A person may be at recommended weight for height, but be overfat.

This fallacy stems from the misconception that all body weight is the same. Fat weight and lean body weight are components of total body weight. Emphasis should be placed on the reduction of excess fat. Redistribution of fat or lean tissue is not possible.

8. *Exercising at high intensity will result in a greater expenditure of calories and a faster rate of weight loss.*

It is true that more intense aerobic exercise produces a greater caloric expenditure per minute when compared to less intensive aerobic exercise. However, the duration of aerobic exercise is the most important variable of caloric expenditure. More intense exercise tends to result in unnecessary fatigue, reduced duration of exercise, delayed onset muscle soreness, higher injury rate, a negative exercise experience and cessation of the exercise program. Exercise of moderate intensity (even exercise of light intensity for the first few weeks) is more likely to result in long term success and attainment of the many physiological and psychological benefits which may result from regular exercise.

9. *Exercise of low intensity will result in greater fat metabolism during exercise and, therefore, a faster, more efficient weight loss.*

This fallacy is relatively new. It originates from the well-established principle that greater fat metabolism takes place during work of low intensity and greater carbohydrate metabolism takes place during work of higher intensity.

The human body utilizes two primary fuels, fat and carbohydrate. We can store much fat and very little carbohydrate. A person at recommended weight may have 25 to 30 pounds of body fat. Each pound contains approximately 3,500 calories which is enough fuel for 35 miles of jogging or 100 miles of cycling. Only about one pound of carbohydrate, which contains less than half the calories of fat, is typically found in the human body. Carbohydrate is an important fuel and, because little is stored, most of our caloric requirement should come from carbohydrate.

Fat and carbohydrate can be conceptualized as being stored in two separate fuel compartments. During both resting and exercise metabolism, fuel is obtained from these two compartments. These fuel stores continue to be drawn upon until replenished by the next meal. As long as the diet contains adequate carbohydrate, the small amount found in the body will remain relatively constant in the long term. Therefore, as long as muscle mass is not being used for fuel, a caloric deficit should result in a reduction of the body's fat stores regardless of the type of fuel used during exercise. Remember that exercise represents a small portion of total daily caloric expenditure and that fat is an important fuel of resting metabolism. As long as aerobic exercise helps to create a caloric deficit and resting metabolism is not depressed by caloric deprivation, a reduction of body fat will take place.

There appears to be no scientific evidence that the type of fuel (fat or carbohydrate) used during exercise influences weight loss or body composition. In the long term, the reduction of body fat is a function of the balance between caloric intake and expenditure.

10. *A weight gain of 3 pounds in a weekend is possible, especially if exercise is not performed.*

This concept can be true or false depending upon the interpretation. It is certainly possible to gain 3 pounds in a day or two. Body fluids have weight and can vary remarkably, depending on a number of factors including nutrition and exercise. However, it is very unlikely that someone could gain 3 pounds of fat in a weekend. To gain 3 pounds of fat, at least 10,500 *extra* calories would have to be consumed, that is, the consumption of 10,500 more calories than are necessary to maintain weight would be required. Such caloric intake is not likely.

11. *Drinking six to eight glasses of water per day or using a water-reducing pill, helps to flush fat from the body.*

Statements related to this concept are made frequently in the weight-loss and exercise industries. The consumption of large amounts of water or the use of diuretics does not cause fat to leave the body by way of urine, feces or sweat. Generally speaking, body fat is used as a fuel when fewer calories are consumed than expended.

12. *Ketones in the urine provide evidence of rapid fat metabolism and a rapid rate of fat loss.*

The staff of some weight-loss programs expect to find chemicals known as ketones in the urine of their participants. The presence of ketones indicates that an individual is adhering to the very low-carbohydrate diet utilized in the weight-loss program. Ketosis (the presence of ketones) indicates that a fuel crisis may exist in the body. As a result of inadequate dietary carbohydrate, protein (muscle mass) is degraded to make new carbohydrate. Therefore, the lean mass is diminished. *Resting metabolism decreases in response to the low calorie, low-carbohydrate diet.* Stored fat is rapidly mobilized, though not rapidly metabolized, in response to the lack of carbohydrate. The mobilization of fat is merely the release of fat from the adipose cells into the blood, not the burning of fat fuel. As fat is mobilized, the liver converts some of the excess fat to ketones which the body can eventually use in a limited way as a carbohydrate substitute. If ketones accumulate to high levels, a severe, life-threatening condition known as ketoacidosis can result. During ketosis, *weight* loss, not necessarily *fat* loss, may be rapid. Ketosis should not occur in a program of body fat reduction.

Determining Percent of Calories from Fat

Foodstuff	Calories
Carbohydrate	4 Calories/gram
Protein	4 Calories/gram
Fat	9 Calories/gram

	Jay's Potato Chips	Mr. Turkey Skinless Turkey Breast	Mr. Turkey Turkey Bologna
Calories	150	104	225
Protein	2g	21g	13g
Carbohydrate	14g	0.5g	.3g
Fat	10g	2g	19g
Fat %	90/150=60%	18/104=17%	171/225=76%
Category	IV	I	IV

Category	Fraction of Calories From Fat	Recommendations
I	less than 1/5 (20% or less)	Highly recommended
II	1/5 to 1/3 (21%–32%)	Recommended, but consider better choices as % of calories from fat approaches 30
III	1/3 to 1/2 (33%–50%)	Limit consumption
IV	Over 1/2 (51% or more)	Consume very infrequently

Category I foods contain no more than 2 grams of fat per 100 calories.
If individuals can average 20% (or less) of all calories in the form of fat, the diet is considered to be excellent relative to fat content.

Chapter Summary

- Habits of nutrition and exercise influence body composition and appearance.
- Changes in the amount of stored body fat are determined by the energy balance equation.
- Fat contains more than twice the calories of other nutrients.
- Americans typically consume too much dietary fat.
- The high-fat diet is associated with an increased risk for heart attack, stroke, cancer and obesity.
- While all fats are high in calories, saturated fat is associated with cardiovascular disease.
- The best method to determine the percent of fat in food is percent of calories, not percent by weight or percent by volume.
- For a given number of calories, more food can be consumed from a high-carbohydrate, low-fat selection than from a choice which is high in fat.
- Consumption of saturated fat is the most important dietary factor which influences blood cholesterol. Consumption of dietary cholesterol is much less important.
- It is desirable to limit total dietary fat to 18% of total caloric intake.
- The Set Point Theory suggests that there is a mechanism in the brain which determines the amount of fat that is stored in the body. Lifestyle factors may influence the set point.
- Heredity plays a role in determining the degree of difficulty in maintaining or achieving recommended weight.
- Even weight-loss diets should contain adequate carbohydrate.
- Ketones in the urine suggest that inadequate carbohydrate is available for fuel.
- The desirable rate of weight loss is one-half to one pound per week.
- The presence of excess body fat is an indication that permanent changes in lifestyle are needed.
- The best weight-loss program is one which involves a lifetime commitment to lifestyle change.
- Aerobic exercise is an essential component of a weight-loss program which is likely to be successful in the long term.

Closing Commentary

The concepts contained in this book have been selected and developed through years of observation of the exercise industry and through preparation of lectures presented over the years to my health science and exercise science classes at Oakland University. One of the most rewarding aspects of teaching is the gratitude expressed by students who have learned how to take positive steps to effectively improve the quality of their lives. I hope that readers of this book will have been helped in a similar manner.

To those who strive to improve in the leading or teaching of exercise and other health-related matters, I wish you good luck and good health and hope that you have found something in this guide to help you along your way.

Rick DeLorme

Fitness and Fallacies Self-Test

True False

☐ ☐ 1. Fifteen minutes of regular aerobic exercise twice per week is adequate to develop reasonably good fitness.

☐ ☐ 2. For general fitness and health, aerobic exercise should be done every day.

☐ ☐ 3. If an exercise causes at least some discomfort, it's probably doing some good.

☐ ☐ 4. Most undesirable body contours are due to poorly toned muscles.

☐ ☐ 5. Toning exercises help to firm and slenderize flabby body regions such as abdomen, thighs, hips and upper arms.

☐ ☐ 6. One-half or more of all people who lose weight through a weight loss diet are able to keep the weight off.

☐ ☐ 7. A weight control plan should be a plan which can be maintained for a life-time, not only a few weeks or months.

☐ ☐ 8. A good weight loss diet should contain little or no carbohydrate.

☐ ☐ 9. Regular aerobic exercise is not an essential component of a weight reduction program.

☐ ☐ 10. Generally speaking, weight loss of 3–7 lbs per week has few, if any, negative consequences.

☐ ☐ 11. The factor most associated with becoming overweight in adulthood is overeating.

☐ ☐ 12. Saturated fat is found only in animal products.

☐ ☐ 13. Cholesterol may be found in animal or plant products.

☐ ☐ 14. Cholesterol in the human body is a harmful substance with no beneficial function.

☐ ☐ 15. If one consumes no cholesterol, there would eventually be none in the blood.

☐ ☐ 16. The best way to reduce blood cholesterol is to greatly reduce or eliminate cholesterol from the diet.

☐ ☐ 17. Foods which are advertised to contain no cholesterol are preferred for reasons of health to those that do contain cholesterol.

☐ ☐ 18. A high protein diet promotes good health and a more attractive body.

☐ ☐ 19. Vegetarians are often not as healthy and often not as energetic as people who eat meat.

☐ ☐ 20. For health reasons, foods which contain vegetable shortening should be preferred to foods which contain animal fat.

True	False		
☐	☐	21.	Most athletes, especially body builders, would benefit from a protein supplement.
☐	☐	22.	Sugary foods consumed immediately before exercise provide quick energy for exercise.
☐	☐	23.	Foods fried in vegetable shortening have fewer calories than foods fried in the same amount of animal fat.
☐	☐	24.	Starchy foods tend to be higher in calories than other foods and therefore tend to be more fattening.
☐	☐	25.	Most Americans don't get enough protein in the diet.

Key: Except for number 7, all are false.

Rick DeLorme, M.A., M.S., is the Assistant Director of the Meadow Brook Health Enhancement Institute at Oakland University, Rochester, Michigan. He is also an Instructor of Exercise Science in Oakland University's School of Health Sciences. In addition to Rick's work in health promotion and disease prevention at the Institute, he supervises the leadership of the Institutès exercise programs. He has directed annual symposia for exercise instructors and other interested individuals. As *Fitness and Fallacies* suggests, Rick has taken an interest in consumer issues related to the exercise industry. Rick's M.A. is in teaching and his M.S. is in exercise science, both from Oakland University.

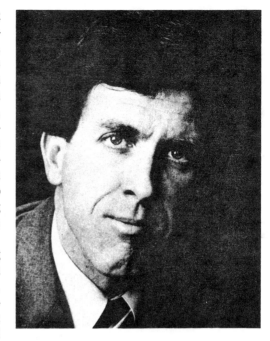

Rick's exercise interests include running and cycling. In eleven years of running, more than 150 competitive events, including four marathons, have been completed. Rick has also directed nearly twenty competitive road runs. Over the past few years, Rick has annually logged one thousand miles of running, through in some years he has run more than two thousand. During winter weather dance-exercise is sometimes substituted. Rick has been involved with cycling since 1974, however, in recent years he has become an enthusiast annually logging more than four thousand miles. Rick's favorite cycling is performance touring along the lake shores and wooded hills on the back roads of northern Michigan. To complete his fitness program, Rick includes resistance training in the Institute's weight room.

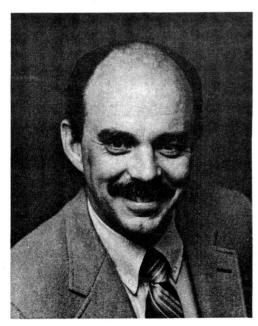

Fred W. Stransky, Ph.D., is the director of the Meadow Brook Health Enhancement Institute and Associate Dean for Health Sciences at Oakland University. He helped to initiate some of the earliest programs in primary and secondary disease prevention in the nation. He lectures regularly on many aspects of health enhancement. His Ph.D. is in Movement Sciences from Florida State University.

Fred was an offensive lineman for the University of Miami in Coral Gables, Florida. Because of his interest in athletics, he pursued a career in exercise physiology. After receiving his Ph.D., he became an avid jogger and lost fifty pounds of his former playing weight. Among other accomplishments, his training led to successful competition in the Boston Marathon. Currently, Fred jogs twenty-five miles per week and participates in a resistance exercise program.